A Dietitian's Dozen Fat-Loss Tips

Paul J. Salter

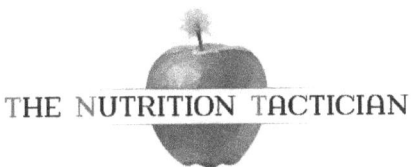

THE NUTRITION TACTICIAN

Published by Createspace, a DBA of On-Demand Publishing, LLC.

Printed in the United States of America

First Printing, 2017

ISBN-13: 978-1542640961

ISBN-10: 1542640962

My goal is to provide you with the information and tools you need to eat healthily and confidently for life.

I hope this books serves you well.

TABLE OF CONTENTS

Hey there,

I'm Paul Salter, Registered Dietitian and founder of the education-driven brands The Nutrition Tactician and TNT University.

The past few years, I've helped more than 600 people 1:1 transform their lives, while collectively losing thousands of pounds of body fat. I've worked with a diverse group of people, including first-time dieters, full-time parents, high-level CrossFit competitors, elite powerlifters and bodybuilders, as well as Collegiate, Professional, and Olympic athletes. I currently serve as a Sports Nutrition Consultant for Renaissance Periodization and as the Nutrition Editor for Bodybuilding.com.

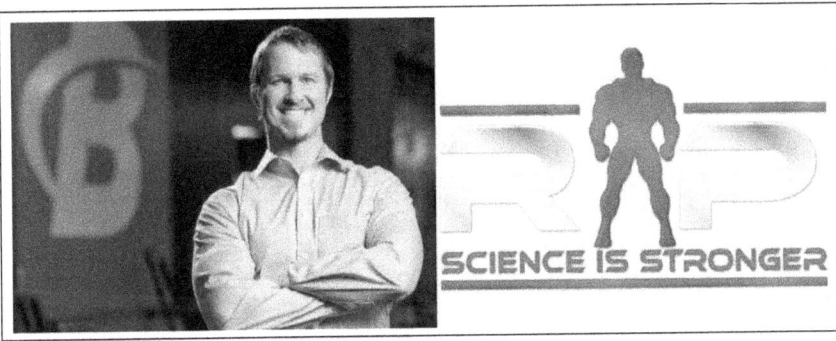

Thank you for taking the time to read this book – I am confident it will serve you well.

This book is a collection of the most effective strategies I have used to help thousands of people master the most fundamental part of weight loss – finding a sustainable approach to nutrition that works and lasts a lifetime.

Thanks again for reading, I hope you enjoy it.

Paul J. Salter

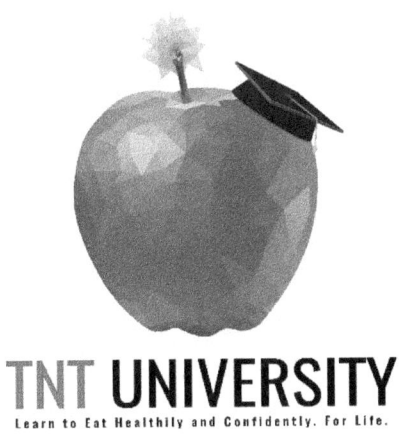

TNT UNIVERSITY

Learn to Eat Healthily and Confidently. For Life.

WHAT THIS BOOK IS NOT...

This book is NOT a diet plan.

It will not detail how to set up an individualized nutrition plan to help you lose weight.

Please do not think that once you finish this book you'll have a precise meal plan and daily calorie goal to begin a diet. That's not the case. If you're at a loss regarding how to implement the strategies you learn, or where to start, please visit please visit www.nutritiontactician.com/coaching to see if 1:1 coaching is right for you.

WHAT THIS BOOK IS...

This book is a collection of strategies I have found to be the most effective in helping hundreds of people lose weight and keep it off. The twelve tips recommended and described in this book are aimed at fighting hunger during a diet, which ultimately will help you make the progress you desire. If you can stay on plan, and have at least a decent approach to weight loss, you can make staggering body composition changes in a rather short amount of time.

Setting the Stage...

Starting a diet is relatively easy.

A combination of eating less and consistently moving more can jump start weight loss. However, completing a diet, well, that's a different story. The first couple of weeks are smooth. Hunger may say "hello" every now and then, but it's manageable. And hey, the weight is coming off, so all is going to plan.

But before long, hunger and fatigue become more frequent and eventually cravings become consistent. Within a few weeks, these two become overwhelming, and ultimately you reach the point of breaking your nutrition plan in favor of something higher in calories. And although some can regain focus (at least for a short while), many aren't so fortunate.

You can lose weight with a low-carb, high-carb, intermittent fasting, or even a high-fat diet approach. But regardless of the dietary set-up you use, one factor remains the same—hunger will be present. And if you're unable to stick to your plan, you will not lose weight. And, well, that just stinks because that's your goal and you've likely invested a lot of time, tears, and energy into this goal. And maybe even some money!

The number one reason a diet fails is lack of adherence. And if we peek behind the gift-wrapped appearance of the ease of dietary adherence, we can see the true struggles: regular hunger, frequent fatigue, and consistent cravings.

It's inevitable. And the longer your diet, the more prominent each becomes. Once you learn to make one or more of these twelve tips routine, however, you'll be able to conquer your next (or current) diet and finally achieve the health and body you've been working for.

I'm excited for you – so get reading!

Note: There are several research studies cited in this book (denoted by a superscript where necessary). For ease of reading, the complete list of references broken down by chapter can be found at the end of this book.

THE GOLDEN RULE OF WEIGHT LOSS

Your weight change is dictated by the relationship between the number of calories you take in and the number of calories you burn.

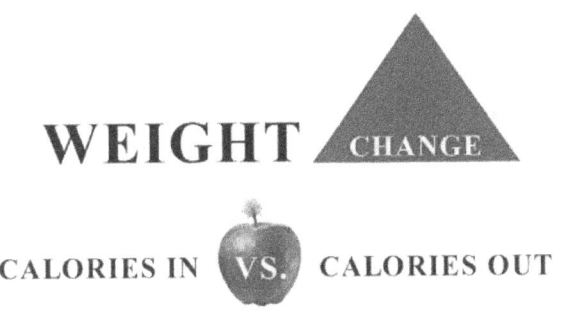

If you take in fewer calories than you burn, you'll lose weight. Conversely, if you take in more calories than you burn, you'll gain weight.

There's no way around this.

When you embark on a diet you begin eating fewer calories than you're burning--if not, you're doing it wrong! Unfortunately, your body views this caloric deficit as a stress; thus, innate survival mechanisms are triggered to return your body back to a weight at which it feels comfortable. This is known as your body fat set point*, or simply, its comfort zone.

Note: Your body fat set point is a range—not one distinct number. For instance, you may fluctuate between 154 – 162 pounds, but getting below 154 pounds is a real struggle because it's the lower end of your body's comfort zone.

These changes (or adaptations) manifest in the form of hunger, fatigue, and an overall decrease in the number of calories you burn each day. The collective effort is to rid the calorie deficit you've created, which, if you remember, is necessary to lose weight.

Dieting isn't Easy

You can have the most positive outlook in the world and a great [diet] plan in place, but hunger and fatigue will still be present. To be honest, this will occur quite often, especially the longer you diet. But by recognizing this, and applying what you learn in this book, your psychological outlook will change and you can prepare accordingly to minimize the effect of diet-induced adaptations.

Without further ado, I present to you a Dietitian's Dozen Fat-Loss Tips.

Enjoy!

Note: These tips are not written in any particular order. Unless you count the fact that I really like protein, so I was eager to jump right in.

CHAPTER 1: PRIORITIZE PROTEIN

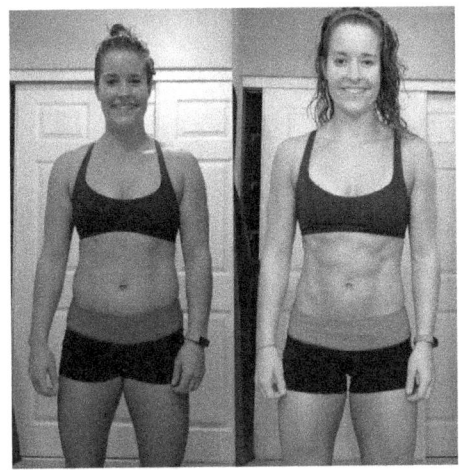

Kaitlin lost 21 pounds in 13 weeks!

You are aware of protein for its role in promoting muscle repair and growth. However, what you may not realize is that protein lends a strong helping hand to your fat-loss efforts, too.

By prioritizing protein, you can enhance your diet adherence, and ultimately, your success. I know, it sounds crazy that I'm recommending you eat more when you're trying to lose weight, but trust me, this is almost a fool-proof strategy.

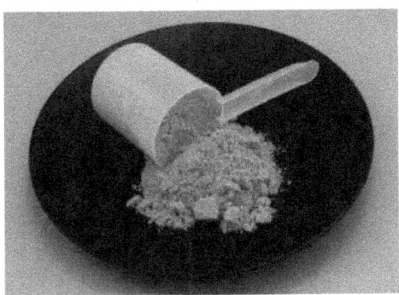

Of course, this doesn't mean you should start shoveling down shakes, and choking down chicken breasts. What it does mean, however, is that if you focus on increasing your protein throughout the day, specifically at each meal, you'll have a much higher rate of success with your weight loss efforts.

Protein positively impacts your fat-loss efforts by:
1. Suppressing hunger
2. Promoting fullness
3. Preserving normal resting metabolic rate
4. Preserving muscle mass

If you recall from the introduction—go back and read if you skipped over it—the relationship between the calories you consume and calories you burn drives weight loss. **You must take in fewer calories than you burn to lose weight**.

There's no way around this.

What's unique about protein is that it significantly impacts both your calorie consumption and your energy expenditure, and it serves as a natural appetite suppressant while simultaneously working to preserve your normal level of calorie expenditure.

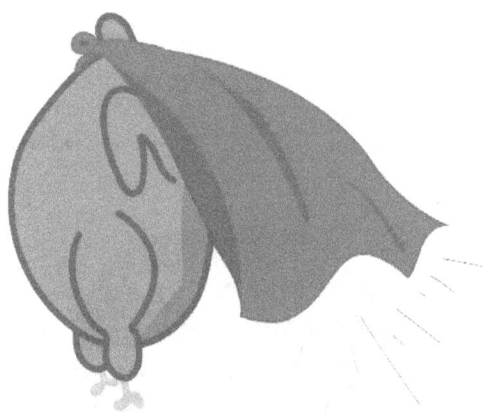

You could say it has super hero-esque qualities.

Impact on Calorie Consumption

In my eyes, the impact protein has on hunger is its most attractive quality.

When you eat protein, it triggers the release of appetite hormones located in your gut. Several of these ultimately work to send signals to your brain to inform it that you're full. Two hormones, cholecystokinin and Peptide YY, do the heavy lifting.

Cholecystokinin - CCK is released from the small intestine and works in two ways to help promote fullness.

1. CCK is believed to play a role in activating the satiety center within the brain. Activation of the satiety center signals fullness and triggers a desire to stop eating. Basically, it's your body's way of yelling at you to "put the fork down!"

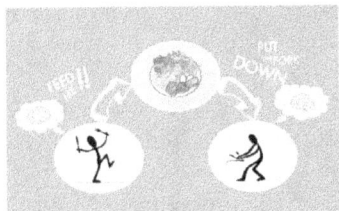

A high-protein meal promotes fullness.

2. Additionally, CCK slows down digestion by delaying the release of food in the stomach to the small intestine. The result of this is an increase in stomach expansion (think of a balloon being filled with water), which is another major satiety signal in and of itself.

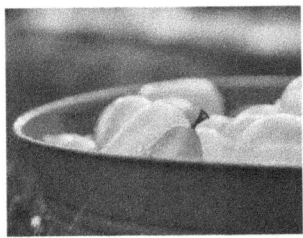

Your stomach expands like a water balloon after a protein rich meal.

Peptide YY- PYY works in a similar manner. It works to delay stomach emptying, thus, promoting satiety via stomach expansion. It has also been shown to act as an appetite suppressant via communication with the hunger center in your brain.

The more protein you eat, the more CCK and peptide YY that are released.[1]

Understanding Energy Expenditure

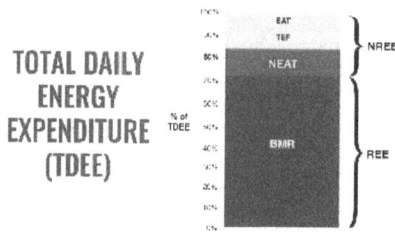

Your **Total Daily Energy Expenditure** (TDEE) refers to the total number of calories you burn throughout a 24-hour period. It's influenced by several factors:

Basal Metabolic Rate- Your basal metabolic rate (BMR) (aka your metabolism) refers to the bare minimum number of calories your body needs to sustain everyday function if it were to be lying in bed for a 24-hour period. These calories are necessary to carry out functions essential to survival, such as breathing, oxygen and blood transport throughout the body, and organ support.

Your metabolism is heavily influenced by your age, size, gender, and amount of muscle mass. It accounts for nearly 70 percent of your TDEE.

Thermic Effect of Food- The thermic effect of food (TEF) refers to the number of calories your body burns to digest, absorb, and distribute nutrients from the food you eat. Believe it or not, eating is an energy-costly process! Thermic effect of foodaccounts for roughly 10 percent of TDEE, which equates to approximately 150 – 200 calories per day for most people.

Exercise and Non-Exercise Activity Thermogenesis- These two terms are exactly what you imagine—the number of calories you burn throughout the day doing exercise and non-exercise activity. Examples of non-exercise activities include walking, carrying out every day activities (think cleaning, cooking, standing), and even the fidgeting or tapping of your foot while you listen to music.

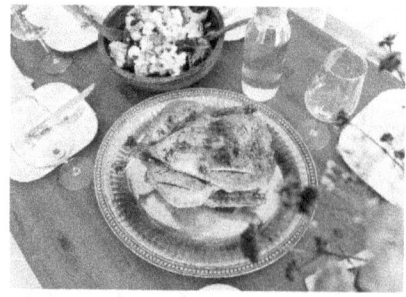

During a diet, each of these components is negatively impacted as your body works to conserve energy and erase the calorie deficit you've created. Fortunately, by **prioritizing protein**, you can help to preserve, or significantly reduce, the negative impact a calorie deficit has on both resting metabolic rate and thermic effect of food.

Prioritizing protein works to maintain the necessary calorie deficit to drive weight loss from multiple angles.

Impact on Energy Expenditure

Your body conserves energy during a diet by reducing your resting metabolic rate (remember, metabolism). A high-protein diet, however, which is characterized by having at least 0.7 grams of protein per pound of body weight, has been shown to maintain metabolic rate during a diet.[2] By **prioritizing protein**, you can preserve a normal level of energy expenditure.

A high-protein diet is equivalent to 105 grams per day for a 150-pound person, and 140 grams per day for a 200-pound person. Chances are that you're eating more – and should be! More on that to come..

Prioritization of protein helps to maintain your hard-earned muscle mass. This is invaluable not only because the end goal of your diet is most likely not to be skinny fat (the result of dieting inappropriately and losing significant muscle), but because muscle mass heavily influences your metabolism.

Support of muscle tissue is energetically costly—your body must work hard (burn more calories) to maintain it. If you have more muscle mass than someone of the same age, gender, height, and weight, the chances are you'll have a greater metabolic rate (this means you require more calories just to maintain your weight).

No matter how optimal your nutrition, training, and supplementation are, a consistent calorie deficit is likely to amount to some degree of muscle loss. With this loss comes a decrease in resting metabolic rate, meaning the calorie deficit you've created further takes a hit. However, the more muscle you lose, the further the reduction in your metabolic rate, which means you must eat even less to see that number on the scale drop.

By **prioritizing protein**, you'll be able to significantly minimize any loss in muscle mass during your fat-loss phase, and ultimately can preserve the necessary calorie deficit. This means you won't have to cut calories as quickly or drastically to reach your goal.

Digestion of protein has a high thermic effect of food relative to carbohydrates and fat.

Protein is very slow to digest because it's quite a challenge for your digestive system. To properly digest and absorb it, your body must expend substantial energy (calories) to do so.

Nutrient	Percent of Calories From Food Burned (%)
Protein	20 – 35
Carbohydrates	5 – 10
Fat	0 - 5

When you eat a meal higher in protein, you burn a greater number of calories compared to if you were to eat the same number of calories from either carbohydrate or fat. For instance, if you were to eat 100 calories of protein from egg whites (nearly 100 percent protein), you could expect to burn 20 – 35 calories digesting, absorbing and distributing these nutrients. If you were to eat 100 calories of carbohydrates from a banana (nearly 100 percent carbohydrates), your body may only expend 5 – 10 calories.

As you can see, **prioritizing protein** at each meal can lead to a significant accumulation of additional energy burned throughout the day.

Consider swapping that afternoon candy bar for a pouch of beef jerky instead. Not only will you burn more calories, but you'll also keep your appetite in check for longer.

What It Means to Prioritize Protein

Now that you have a firm understanding of why it's imperative to **prioritize protein** during your diet, it's time to provide you with the information and tools necessary to execute.

I want you to focus on choosing a high-quality protein source (from the list below) every three to five hours (this means at all meals <u>and</u> snacks).

High-Quality Protein Sources

- Eggs: whites and yolks
- Chicken breast (without skin)
- Turkey breast (without skin)
- Ground meats: chicken/turkey/beef (90/10 or leaner)
- Beef: flank steak, steak sirloin, filet mignon, top and bottom round
- Pork: pork tenderloin, ham, Canadian bacon
- Game meats: bison, elk, deer (venison)
- Lean Jerky: beef, turkey, bison, elk, deer, salmon
- Lean deli meat: chicken, turkey, ham, roast beef
- Dairy: Greek yogurt, cottage cheese, milk, cheese
- Fish: salmon, tuna, mackerel, cod, tilapia, etc.
- Seafood: shrimp, oysters, scallops, mussels, etc.
- Plant-based protein: soy, tofu, quinoa
- Protein powder: whey, casein, beef, soy, complete vegetable protein

Every three to five hours, strive for 25 – 35 grams of protein from the sources above.

IMPORTANT: The trace amount of protein found in your carbohydrate or fat sources at your meal should NOT contribute to your protein total. For example, do not count the five grams of protein found in a ½-cup serving of oatmeal towards your meal total.

Why?
Plant protein (the protein found in grains, nuts, seeds, vegetables, beans, and legumes) is incomplete, meaning it doesn't contain all nine essential amino acids necessary to optimize muscle repair and growth. Without all nine essential amino acids, a protein's function is sub-optimal.

You absolutely can and should still eat sources of plant protein, however, they shouldn't be the lone source of protein at your meal. If you're choosing not to have animal protein, for whatever reason, you should pair two or more incomplete protein sources together to form a complementary protein.

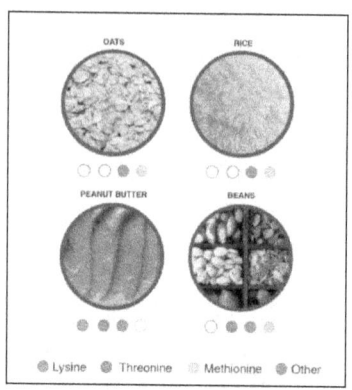

Two common complementary protein pairings include rice and beans,
as well as oats and peanut butter.

This means combining a plant protein that is lacking a particular amino acid(s) with one that has that missing amino acid(s) to achieve all nine essential amino acids at the meal. Examples include pairing rice and beans, peanut butter and whole grain bread, or pita bread and hummus.

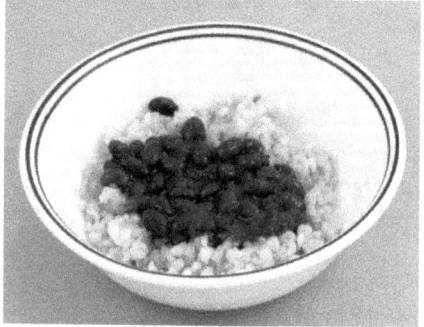

Note: Discussing vegetarian and vegan protein needs and sources is outside the scope of this book, however, feel free to reach out to me with any specific questions you have. You can contact me at paul@nutritiontactician.com.

Chapter 1 Recap

- Protein positively impacts both sides of the weight loss equation.

- Protein promotes fullness by triggering the release of several gut hormones that send satiety signals to the brain and by also slowing down digestion.

- Protein is very costly (in terms of calories) to digest. Your body burns more energy (calories) digesting, absorbing, and distributing calories (Thermic Effect of Food) from protein compared to either carbohydrates or fat.

- Protein helps to preserve your metabolic rate and muscle mass, which has a tremendous impact on your metabolic rate.

- Most will benefit from striving for 25 – 35 grams of high-quality protein (see list of sources above) every 3 – 5 hours.

CHAPTER 2: CHOOSE CARBOHYDRATES HIGH IN FIBER

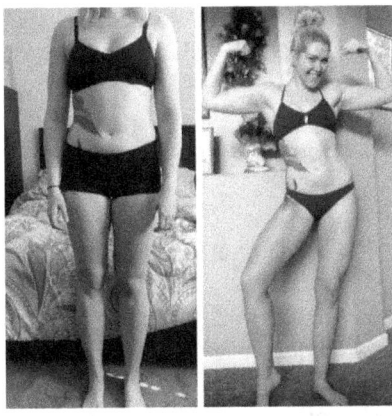

Adrianna lost 13 pounds in 12 weeks!

Carbohydrates get called a lot of names.

"Tasty."

"Delicious."

"Fattening."

"The Devil."

It's unfortunate that so much love, hatred, and uncertainty revolves around the word "carbs." At the root of it, they're your body's primary energy source. So, you kind of *need* them...

And yes, you even need them when embarking on a fat-loss phase.

But the type of carbohydrate you choose matters. To enhance energy, exercise performance, satiety, and ultimately the success of your diet, **choose carbohydrates high in fiber**.

Note: High-fiber carbohydrates should be your primary choice regardless of your nutrition goal—the health benefits are invaluable. During a diet, however, high-fiber carbohydrates become even more important because they help to enhance energy and suppress appetite between meals.This is crucial considering diets often fail due to fatigue and overwhelming hunger.

Focus on Fibrous Carbohydrates

Fiber is a type of carbohydrate.
What's unique about fiber, however, is that it's a dense structure that is indigestible by the human body. It literally passes through your digestive system nearly unscathed. Along the way, it takes up water, which further slows the digestive process by increasing the bulk of the stomach contents that move through your digestive tract.

This profound impact has significant carry over to effect both appetite and energy levels.

The Ripple Effect of Slow Digestion

The bulking of food through water absorption (that's promoted by a high-fiber meal) leads to more space being taken up in your stomach. This is great news when you're striving to achieve fullness because your stomach is a "volume counter," rather than a "calorie counter."

The more space you take up with food or fluids, the fuller you feel.[1]Technically, this is called satiety. It occurs due to an accumulation of substantial food in the stomach, which leads to stretching of the stomach wall and a strong signal being sent to your brain indicating fullness.

This impact on digestion has a ripple effect and positively influences blood glucose and insulin levels, too. Because of slowed digestion, glucose enters the blood at a slower rate, which means less insulin is needed to shuttle glucose into storage.

Together, this leads to more stable blood glucose levels, which is highly desirable considering that a rapid spike, followed by a reduction, in blood glucose can lead to early onset hanger and fatigue shortly after a meal. Ultimately, slower digestion correlates with more stable blood glucose levels and more stable energy levels in between meals.

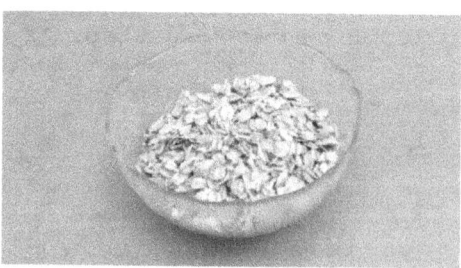

High-Fiber Carbs ↓Hunger ↓Insulin ↑Energy

A low-fiber carbohydrate, on the other hand, digests quickly. As you can imagine, this leads to a spike in blood glucose and surge in insulin levels. The sudden spike in blood glucose often leads to overcompensation of insulin production causing a quick return to baseline blood glucose levels, which will soon decrease even further.

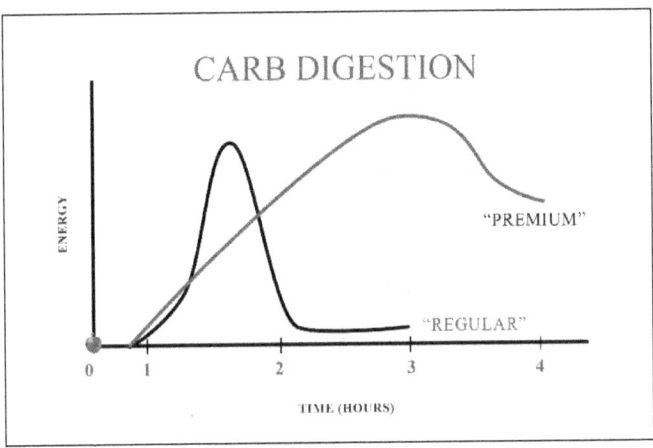

A premium carbohydrate is one that's high in fiber and rich in essential nutrients.

It's no wonder you can plow through a whole box of your favorite cereal but struggle to finish a second serving of broccoli. The high-fiber nature of the broccoli takes up more space in your stomach, which sends signals to your brain to put down the fork.

Low blood glucose levels lead to fatigue and hunger—a dieter's worst nightmare, especially when this occurs shortly after eating.

Choosing High-Fiber Carbohydrates

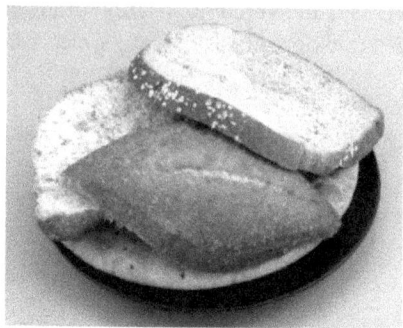

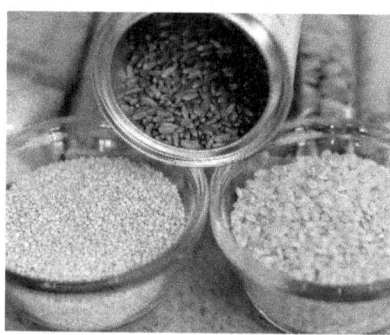

High-Fiber Carbohydrates

- Whole-grain bread, wraps, bagels, and pasta
- Brown and wild rice
- Quinoa
- Oats
- Barley
- Beans and legumes
- High-fiber cereal (Cheerios, Wheaties, Fiber One, Kashi Go Lean Crunch)
- Popcorn
- Fruit
- Vegetables

Now that you have a firm understanding of why it's imperative to **choose high-fiber carbohydrates** during your diet, it's time to provide you with the information and tools necessary to execute a workable plan.

There are two strategies that I recommend using to ensure you **choose a high-fiber carbohydrate**:

1. **Select Dark Brown Carbohydrates**- Okay, this doesn't always work, but it's an excellent starting point. Those darker carbohydrates that are more brown in color tend to be much higher in fiber than those sources that are pale or whitish-yellow in color. Examples include selecting brown rice over white rice, whole-wheat pasta in place of white pasta, or any whole grain bread, wrap, or bagel, in favor of a white option.

2. **Use the 6:1 Rule**- The above rule works well with most of your typical "meal" foods, however, snack foods, such as bars, crackers, chips, and more are a bit trickier to navigate. That's where the 6:1 rule comes into play.

   a. Find the nutrition label of your item of interest.
   b. Find the number of total carbohydrates (grams).
   c. Find the number of total/dietary fiber (grams).
   d. Divide total carbohydrates by total/dietary fiber. This will leave you with a ratio.

Nutrition Facts

Serving Size	1 1/4 Cup (58g)

Amount Per Serving

Calories 180	Calories from Fat 15

	% Daily Value*
Total Fat 2g	3%
Saturated Fat 0g	0%
Trans Fat 0g	
Polyunsaturated Fat 1g	
Monounsaturated Fat 0g	
Cholesterol 0mg	0%
Sodium 115mg	5%
Pot~~assium~~	11%
Total Carbohydrate 40g	1~~3~~%
Dietary Fiber 13g	52%
Soluble Fiber 1g	
Insoluble Fiber 12g	
Sugars 8g	
Protein 12g	17%

Example: Total Carbohydrates = 40 g
Dietary Fiber = 13 g
Ratio = 40 g / 13 g = ~3:1 ratio

The lower the ratio of the food item, the higher the fiber per serving, and more likely it is to contain less sugar too. The result: slow digestion and long-lasting energy (and fullness) for the hours to come!

Your goal is to find an item with a low ratio, **aiming for 6:1 or lower**. This indicates that the food has more fiber per serving, thus, a more positive impact on energy levels and appetite. Not every healthy snack option will have a 6:1 ratio but when comparing a few of your favorite snacks or brands, selecting the one with the lower ratio will be your best bet. If you can't find your favorite snack at a ratio of 12:1 or lower, opt for something different.

The 6:1 strategy works great with cereals, breads, wraps, and bagels, too!

And lastly, as icing on the cake, if you're ever unsure, you can triple confirm that you have selected a premium, high-fiber carbohydrate by checking the ingredients list. The first ingredient—which is the one added in the highest amount—should be a whole-grain product, which indicates it's high in fiber. Such examples include whole-wheat flour, oats, brown rice, quinoa, etc. Not white, or refined flour, or any other sugary-sounding name. If you can't pronounce it, the chances are it's not a whole grain.

If you want to learn everything you need to know about carbohydrates, sign up for my online video course entitled "Carbohydrate Confidence" today! Visit www.courses.nutritiontactician.com to get started.

Chapter 2 Recap:

- Fiber is an indigestible starch that slows digestion and pulls water into the gut. Both of these properties increase satiety.

- The delay in digestion because of choosing a high-fiber carbohydrate has a positive impact on blood glucose and energy levels, as well as your appetite.

- Low-fiber carbohydrates digest quickly and lead to a quick spike and drop in both blood glucose and insulin levels. This has a negative impact on energy and appetite, and over time, can have a significant impact on your health, too.

- Two simple strategies to ensure you're choosing a high-fiber carbohydrate include:

    o Choose darker, browner carbohydrates.

    o Utilize the 6:1 strategy as detailed above.

- If you want to know everything you need to know about carbohydrates, sign up for my "Carbohydrate Confidence" course today!

CHAPTER 3: EAT VEGETABLES WITH EACH MEAL

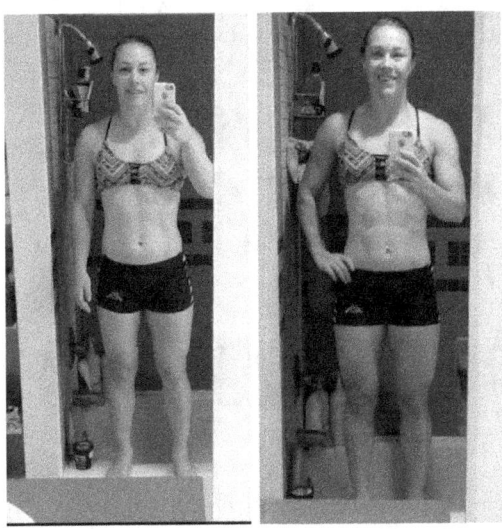

Emily lost 8 pounds in 10 weeks to make weight for her Olympic Weightlifting meets.
She set new PRs left and right and qualified for multiple elite competitions in 2017.

Seriously.

Even at breakfast and your bed time snack.

You're foolish for skimping on vegetables when you're not dieting, but even more foolish when you are. Vegetables not only provide a bounty of health benefits, but also numerous advantages that will help you stick to your diet.

So yes, **eat vegetables with each meal**.

The Bounty of Health Benefits

Vegetables are rich in essential vitamins and minerals, antioxidants, phytochemicals, and are loaded with fiber and water. The latter two have a profound impact on keeping hunger in check, which we'll discuss in a second. But first, I want to acknowledge the health-specific benefits.

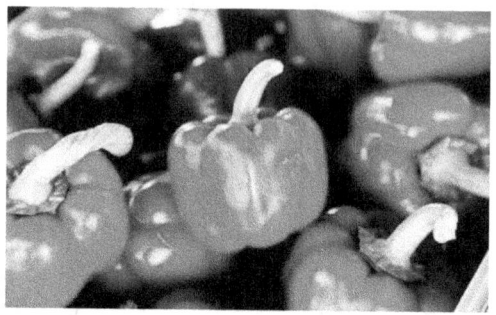

Vegetables provide the complete package!

Vitamins and minerals play an integral role in all bodily functions aimed at helping you survive and thrive. They play a crucial role in energy production, immune function, growth, repair, development, skin health, cognitive function, and memory.

Antioxidants and phytochemicals further bolster health by providing an additional layer of protective benefit. These molecules have even been shown to play a major role in slowing the aging process, bolstering immune function, and lessening your chance for developing various diseases and cancers.

What more do you need to start eating vegetables?

Go ahead and grab a handful of carrots before you read any further.

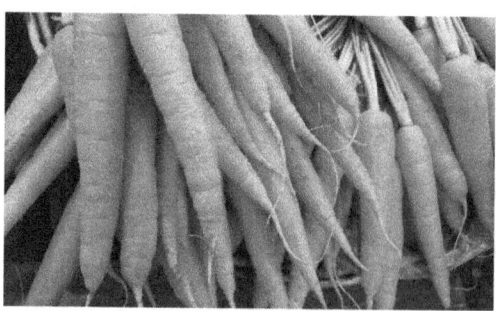

Carrots taste great raw, but even better (and sweeter) when steamed or roasted.

A Dieter's Best Friend

I was serious about the carrots...

Vegetables are an excellent source of fiber. Furthermore, they're also very high in water—most are composed of over 90 percent!

The combination of fiber and water attacks hunger head on by slowing digestion and taking up a lot of space in your stomach (at a very low calorie cost).

Remember, your stomach is a volume counter. By filling it with a large amount of high-fiber, high-water foods, you'll begin to feel full quickly. And what further differentiates vegetables from other high-fiber carbohydrates is their **very low calorie per** bite **ratio**!

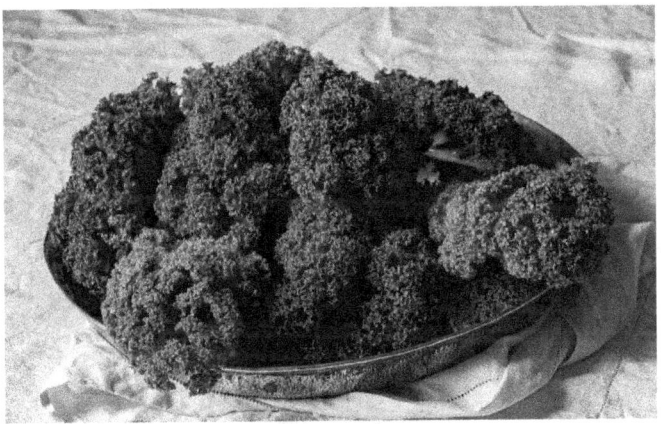

A typical serving of vegetables has between 10 – 50 calories, whereas a serving of brown rice or oats has well over 100 calories per serving.

By stockpiling your plate with vegetables, you allow yourself the opportunity to eat a large volume of food, with little caloric consequence. This is an invaluable strategy to curtail hunger because of the miniscule calorie impact derived from achieving a sense of physical and mental satiety.

How to Eat More Vegetables

If everyone loved vegetables I probably wouldn't have dedicated an entire chapter of this book to them. The main reason most individuals don't eat vegetables, despite the many health and fat-loss benefits they offer, is because of their "vegetable" taste.

Many would describe vegetables, as bland, bitter,or even downright disgusting.

If you're one who doesn't enjoy vegetables, fear not—I have many strategies you can use to increase the amount you eat to reap their innumerable benefits mentioned above. And once you start incorporating these strategies, you may find that you begin to enjoy them...and even crave them...but we'll start with baby steps.

1. **Cook Them**- The thought of a raw broccoli floret is a turn off to many, myself included, yet, I love broccoli. But when it's raw, it has a rather bitter taste. Cooking broccoli, however, along with any other vegetable, breaks down the bitter starches into **pleasant tasting sugars**, which brings about a subtle, sweet taste. Consider roasting, steaming, or grilling your vegetables to enhance palatability.

   This works especially well for broccoli, carrots, bell peppers, and zucchini.

2. **Scramble Them**- A savory, fluffy omelet or egg scramble can easily mask the flavor of a handful of vegetables. Consider sautéing peppers, onions, spinach, or broccoli, before adding your eggs to the pan. Throw in a bit of cheese, your favorite seasoning blend, and you'll further elevate the health, taste, and texture of your meal!

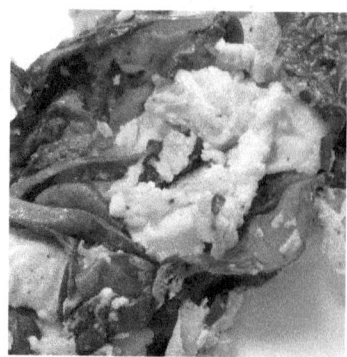

3. **Blend Them**- To further enhance your smoothie, sneak in some spinach! Yes, your smoothie will turn green, however, the spinach taste will be masked by the other ingredients you've added. Consider adding fruit, or your favorite nut butter to the smoothie, as each has a strong flavor that will absolutely crush the light taste spinach provides. Drink up!

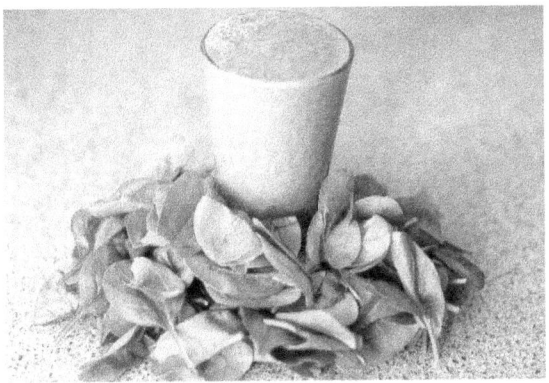

4. **Hide Them**- Sneak a piece—or three—of your favorite dark, leafy green vegetable into your next sandwich. Hidden between two slices of whole grain bread, savory protein (my go-to is lean deli turkey), and creamy cheese (yum, provolone), the vegetable taste will be masked. And for a little extra crunch, try adding bell peppers, cucumbers, onions, or pickles!

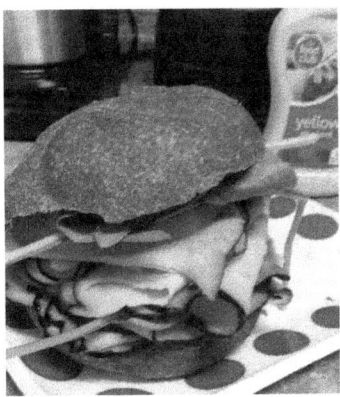

5. **Dress Them**- Hot sauce, dressing, salsa, soy sauce, or low-fat cheese—each is an easy way to add a preferable flavor to your veggies. One of my favorite ways to enjoy steamed broccoli is to layer string cheese across the broccoli once it's done cooking so that the cheese melts all over it. Yum!

6. **Dip Them**- Consider dipping your vegetables into a low-fat spread, hummus, or homemade Greek yogurt concoction. For a healthy Ranch dressing alternative, purchase a Ranch seasoning packet(s) and add (as desired) to low-fat, plain Greek yogurt. Stir, dip, and enjoy! Carrots, cucumbers, celery, and sliced bell peppers pair well.

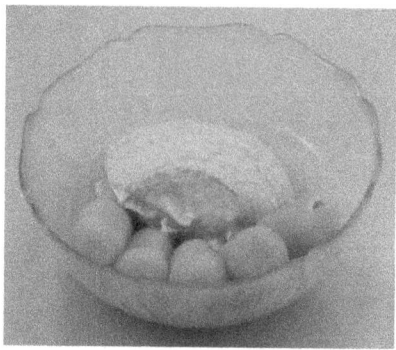

7. **Season Them**- Don't be shy on the seasoning! Add any spice, herb, or seasoning to further elevate the flavor. I never eat veggies without salt and garlic powder.

And lastly, keep this in mind: **Your taste buds change over time**.

Seriously.

Let me tell you a quick story.

When I first became interested in nutrition, I was intrigued by natural bodybuilding. So, I made myself a strict meal plan to follow (we all start somewhere!) to prepare for a competition. Breakfast on day one was an egg white and vegetable omelet, a cup of oatmeal, and a tablespoon of peanut butter.

The omelet was no issue at all—hot sauce and a little ketchup did the trick. The oatmeal and peanut butter however, was a disaster.

Not only was I unable to finish the meal, but I almost threw up...

I did not finish my breakfast that morning...

Fast forward and now peanut butter is my favorite food and I can't remember that last day I went without at least one tablespoon. And peanut butter-oatmeal is one of my favorite meals! Boy how the times (and my taste buds!) have changed.

My point is this: make the effort to make vegetables a part of your daily routine. If you didn't like cauliflower six months ago, try it again. You may find it more palatable this time around. If you don't like it, no big deal. At least now you know and can confirm that. Fortunately, there are many options to choose from.

Chapter 3 Recap:

- Vegetables offer a bounty of health benefits. They're rich in vitamins, minerals, fiber, antioxidants, and phytochemicals. Regardless of your weight goal, vegetables should be a stale in your day.

- Vegetables help fight hunger head-on because they're rich in both water and fiber. Water and fiber each work to take up space in your stomach, which sends satiety signals to your brain.

- There are several strategies you can use to "sneak" vegetables into your day: cook, scramble, blend, hide, dress, dip, and season.

- Your taste buds change over time – give a new vegetable a chance today!

CHAPTER 4: HYDRATE, HYDRATE, HYDRATE

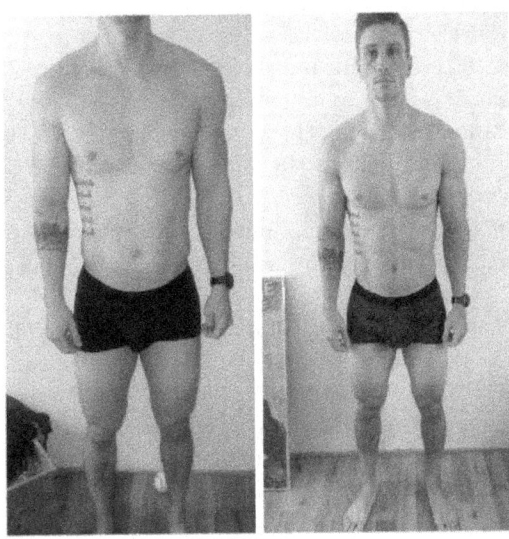

Ross lost 16 pounds in 14 weeks!

When one of my 1:1 clients informs me that they're feeling hungry or fatigued, the first component of their daily routine I address is their hydration habits.

Why?

Because your body is made up of roughly 70 percent water. Even more specifically, your brain is composed of nearly 80 percent, and your muscles 75 percent. As you can imagine, the slightest bit of dehydration can wreak havoc on cognitive and physical performance, as well as your appetite and energy levels.

It's likely that at some point during a diet you will feel hungry and tired. That's inevitable. So, when you are dieting, I advise you to **hydrate, hydrate, hydrate**.

Before I discuss the consequences of dehydration in more detail, it's important to first address the sensation of "thirst" and what it means when you *feel* thirsty.

Understanding the Thirst Mechanism

The "thirst center" of your brain is located within the hypothalamus, which is the region of your brain also responsible for regulating appetite. A complex network of feedback loops throughout the body helps to communicate fluid needs to this region of the brain. This includes in-body sensors that regulate changes in blood volume and pressure, as well as changes in sodium levels. Even the slightest change outside of normal limits can be *felt* in the thirst center.

Translation: Your body closely monitors your hydration status and takes the necessary actions to prompt you to stay hydrated.

Unfortunately, despite the complexity of this mechanism, the thirst sensation is relatively weak.
What I mean by that is when you finally do feel thirsty, you're already dehydrated. So maybe "slow" is a better way to characterize the sensation. Basing your fluid needs on waiting until you *feel* thirsty isn't something I recommend.

In addition, for reasons not yet fully understood, this complex feedback network weakens with age. Thus, it becomes increasingly difficult to recognize thirst before reaching an even greater level of dehydration as you get older.

And even worse, when you're dehydrated, you often mistake this sensation for hunger.

One reason this may occur is because hunger and dehydration have similar signs and symptoms—fatigue, irritability, and lack of focus. Additionally, its plausible to think that the brain recognizes it's in need of water and associates eating with the delivery of fluids (most foods are composed of a large percentage of water). Thus, you begin to *feel* hungry as a survival mechanism to promote fluid intake. And given that it's habitual to consume fluids with meals more often than in between meals this makes sense.

As you can see, thirst is a misunderstood and weak sensation. This is unfortunate considering the strong impact even the slightest bit of dehydration can have on your day, and ultimately, your fat-loss efforts.

But my guess is that your favorite food isn't the nutrient dense, low-calorie carrot, but probably more akin to the calorie-rich vending machine candy bar. If your hydration game is weak, it's likely you're giving in to one too many off-plan treats, which is holding you back from making the fat-loss progress you'd hoped for.

From an exercise standpoint, as little as 2 - 3 percent dehydration can wreak havoc on your physical performance.[1,2]This equates to losing as little as four pounds during an exercise session for a 200-pound individual. And given that sweat rates may be as high as 1.5 – 2.0 liters per hour, a two percent loss in body weight can occur in a flash if proper hydration habits aren't in place.

Signs and symptoms of dehydration include:

- Fatigue
- Headaches
- Lightheadedness
- Dizziness
- Lack of focus
- Irritability
- Muscle cramps
- Increased rating of perceived exertion
- Increased injury risk
- Decreases in strength, power, and endurance
- Slower reaction time

I'm sure you've experienced one or many of these before.

Each one limits your performance, and ultimately decreases the number of calories you burn. This negatively impacts the weight change equation we discussed earlier, and ultimately reduces the calorie deficit you're striving to create to drive fat-loss…

This is not a recipe for success.

Fluids and Fullness

The crux of why you need to focus on hydration is related to the prominent impact fluids have on hunger. As I've discussed already, your stomach is a volume counter, not a calorie counter. Therefore, when you fill it with food or fluids and it begins to stretch, satiety signals are sent to your brain to encourage you to put the fork down.

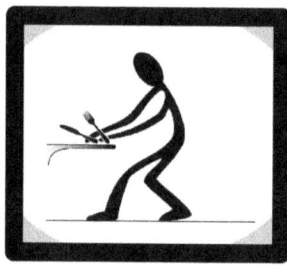

Filling your stomach with fluids sends signals to your brain to make you put the fork down at meals.

Fluids move quickly through the digestive tract, much faster than foods. Thus, they're able to fill your stomach rapidly. This leads to quicker stomach expansion, and **feeling full sooner**. Of even more significance, depending on the fluid you choose—I'm advocating for water most of the time—you're filling your body with zero calories.

Increased fullness without calories? That's a tough combination to beat when on a diet. A desirable situation to be in, to say the least!

How Much Should I Drink?

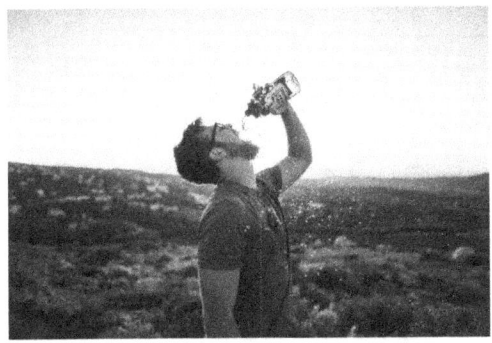

Fluid needs are highly individualized, but yours are most likely higher
than what you're currently doing.

Your fluid needs are largely influenced by your age, size, training habits, climate, and altitude. However, a starting point that works well for all is as follows:

- Women should aim for a minimum of 96 ounces (roughly three liters) per day.

- Men should aim for a minimum of 125 fluid ounces (roughly four liters, or one gallon) per day.

However, these recommendations do not include the increased need for fluids when exercising. **During exercise, strive for an additional 5 – 8 ounces of fluids for every 15 minutes of exercise.** If your workout lasts 60 minutes, you should strive for 20 – 32 ounces of fluids throughout.

Am I Hydrated?

For immediate feedback on your hydration habits, assess the color of your urine.

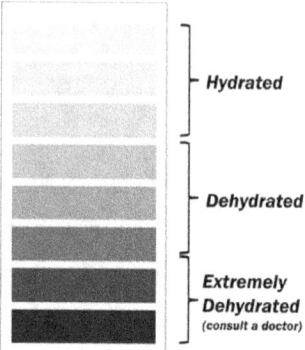

Your urine color is an excellent indicator of your hydration status.

Your urine color should be "light like lemonade," not "dark like apple juice." The former indicates you're well hydrated, whereas the latter is a sign you're in need of fluids stat.

It's worth mentioning that striving for a urine color "clear like water" is less than ideal, and may be as detrimental as being "dark like apple juice." This overhydrated state indicates that you're low on electrolytes, particularly sodium, which is responsible for retaining water in the body. If you notice your urine color is clear, seek out a salty snack(s) and add salt to your next few meals. If it's a common occurrence, consider making salt a regular staple with each meal.

A word of caution: If you find yourself far off from these recommendations, don't try to double, or even triple, your total fluid consumption overnight. You and your bladder will hate me. Instead, gradually work up to these goals. Start with an increase of 8 – 12 ounces per day for 2 – 3 days and continue to gradually increase until you're at your goal.

What Should I Drink?

Water.

Or, at least only calorie-free liquids.

Why?

Liquids digest quickly. Drinking fast-digesting calories is more likely to lead to consumption of far greater calories than you need. This is no Bueno. Plus, water is essential, and free almost everywhere you go.

Aside from water, there are many calorie-free alternatives from which to choose. Coffee, tea, diet sodas, and artificially flavored waters are popular options. Each is primarily composed of water, and contains virtually zero calories, too.

Note: Yes, you can still drink calorie-containing fluids and lose weight. But if sticking to a diet in the past has been a challenge because of persistent hunger, then you may consider focusing on calorie-free options and eating your calories instead.

When Should I Drink?

Right now.

Seriously, take a sip of something before continuing...

Strategies to Enhance Hydration

1. **Carry A Water Bottle Everywhere**- Treat it like you would your wallet or purse—have it on hand in the car, while at your desk, while in meetings, while at the gym, and, of course, at each, and every meal. It should always be in sight so that you're reminded to drink from it.

2. **Invest in a Larger Water Bottle**- Choosing a small water bottle can be a pain when trying to increase your hydration habits because it leaves you feeling as if you need to fill it up every 15 minutes.

    Talk about a turn off.

    You don't have to go to the opposite side of the spectrum and begin carrying a gallon around with you, though there's nothing wrong with that. Instead, opt for a bottle that holds at least 24 ounces to reduce trips to the water fountain.

Advanced Hydration Strategies to Conquer Hunger

1. **Drink upon Waking-** I recommend you drink 12 – 16 ounces immediately upon waking. So, yes, that means you should sleep with your water bottle, or a glass of water, on your night stand!

2. **Pre-Load Meals-** Drink 12 – 16 ounces of water 10 – 15 minutes before each meal. This will lead to you sitting down for your meal less hungry because of the significant amount of fluid taking up space in your stomach.

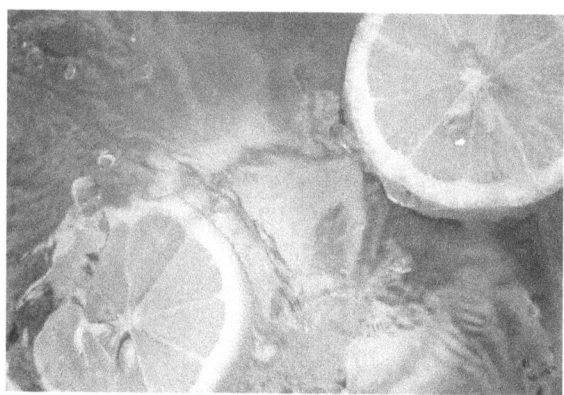

Hydrate, hydrate, hydrate.

3. **Book-End Meals-** Similarly to pre-loading, end each meal with another 12 – 16 ounces of water, to further stretch your stomach and promote fullness.

4. **Choose Carbonated Drinks-** Selecting a (calorie-free) carbonated drink will further help suppress your appetite by taking up even more space in your stomach. That's because these beverages have carbon dioxide added. Instead of just fluid taking up space in your stomach, you now have fluid plus air—a one, two-punch, if you will—to fight hunger head on.

Final Word

The chances are that you'll want to increase your total daily fluid intake after reading this chapter. I recommend grabbing a glass of water before continuing to the next information-packed chapter!

Getting back on track...

By increasing the amount of fluid you drink, the number of trips you make to the bathroom will increase, too. At least, initially. More specifically, you may find yourself waking in the middle of the night once, or twice. Stay patient. Your body will adjust if you remain consistent and gradually increase your intake. If one day you hit 150 total ounces, and the next day 65, and so forth, well, you and your bladder are in for a rough ride.

Chapter 4 Recap:

- Your body is composed largely of water. Dehydration can significantly impact both your cognitive and physical performance, and has a profound impact on your appetite, too.

- Hunger is often the result of dehydration.

- Read the above point again.

- Prioritizing fluids can help to promote fullness because the quick-digesting nature of liquids rapidly expands your stomach, which trigger satiety signals to be sent to your brain. Drinking fluids before, during, after, and in between meals can crush hunger and cravings and keep you on plan.

- The color of your urine reflects your hydration status. Aim for "light like lemonade."

- Women should aim for a minimum of 96 ounces (roughly three liters) per day.

- Men should aim for a minimum of 125 fluid ounces (roughly four liters, or one gallon) per day.

- During exercise, aim to drink an additional 5 – 8 fluid ounces every 15 minutes.

CHAPTER 5: EAT BLAND FOOD

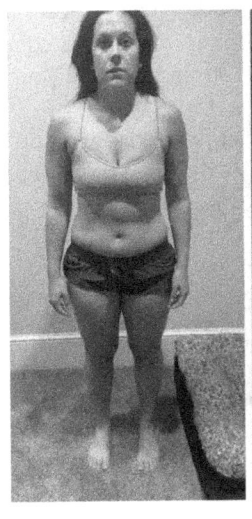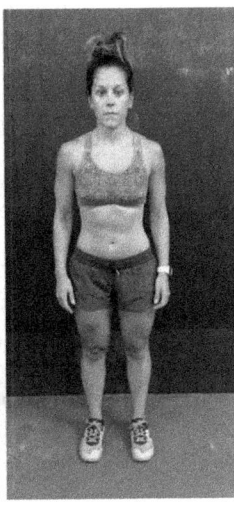

Casey lost 17 pounds in 13 weeks!

Yes, it's possible to eat ice cream and your favorite treats while dieting and to still lose weight. Heck, in most cases, it's encouraged (in moderation, of course).

But when taken too far, extreme flexibility can work against your dieting efforts, rather than for them. This is especially true as you get deeper into a diet, when cravings become a recurrent part of your day.

R.I.P. carbs.

As your diet continues, cravings gradually grow stronger.

At first, they're easy to ignore. Well, easier, at least.
But as you progress further into your diet, you need to pull out a few Nutrition Tactician-recommended strategies to keep them at bay. You chug back a glass of water, and refocus your mind on the task at hand. Eventually, however, you begin to develop the urge to have "just one" spoonful of ice cream. But as soon as that ice cream touches your tongue, it sends your taste buds dancing, and there's no turning back.

Dance Party!

That one spoonful quickly turns into one pint, ultimately negating your hard work for the day, and possibly the past few. Thanks, a lot, Ben and Jerry.

We've both been there.

Remember, dieting is a stress and your body employs every tactic it can to get you to eat more and re-establish a sense of normalcy in its comfort zone. Hunger and intense cravings are one of the most successful tools your body employs.

But what if there was a way to avoid that need for "just one" cookie, scoop of ice cream, or finger of peanut butter? What if you could repress the expected craving signal so strongly that it virtually disappears?

Eat bland food, and you can, and it will.

By **eating bland food**, over and over, it turns out that you can indeed repress a strong desire for anything and everything fluffed with flavor and loaded with calories. And when you're well into a diet, **this becomes invaluable**. Late in the game, your metabolism has significantly slowed and one binge can set you back days, or even a week's, worth of hard work.

> *If you're sick of failing to stick to a diet,*
> *and sick of not having your body reflect the hard work*
> *you're putting in at the gym, then eat bland food.*

What Happens Each Time You Eat Flavorful Food?

It's no secret that the better a food tastes, the more likely you are to eat it. Heck, you'll even drive 30-minutes out of the way on your way home for your favorite ice cream sundae!

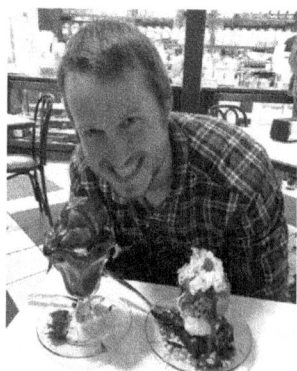

This ice cream spot in Boise wasn't *too* far out of the way

Don't worry, you're not alone.

Rats have been known to push through electric shock and extreme cold to eat a highly palatable pellet despite having just eaten, or, having standard chow readily available.[1,2]

But each time you take a trip to flavor town, you send your taste buds dancing and provide them with a tango of a lifetime. The problem, however, lies in how often you send them dancing. If your dieting approach is too flexible and is one where you work in super sweet, fatty, or flavorful treats often, then your taste buds experience quite a bit of dancing.

And when this occurs, your taste buds will feel as if you've signed them up for daily dance lessons. Or, even dance lessons every few hours! When you forget to drop them off at dance lessons, or have a typical "diet" meal (such as baked tilapia and steamed broccoli), they get feisty. They let your brain know that they haven't danced in what seems like forever. And what ensues is a strong urge for anything and everything that will provide them with an opportunity to dance again.

If only dancing wasn't so expensive (in calories)...

But if you don't let your taste buds dance too often, if at all, during a diet, they're less likely to grow feisty because they don't become accustomed to daily dancing. Instead, they enjoy the dancing as it comes, and remain content in between. This translates to better dietary adherence, and ultimately better progress. Now, that is reason to dance!

Note: If you were unable to keep up with the beat of the music, here's what I am trying to say:

When you eat your favorite foods, your brain is flushed with dopamine. Dopamine is a chemical released in the brain that is associated with feelings of reward and pleasure. It's the same chemical that fuels the rush drug users feel immediately after using, and it has a major impact on addiction. This same rush has been shown to occur with food, too, as dopamine plays a large role in food-reinforcing behaviors and food reward.[3,4]

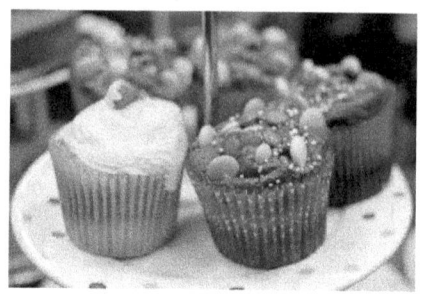

High-sugar foods create a similar release in dopamine that drug users feel when suffering from addiction.

Once the flavorful food touches your tongue, you enter a brief state of euphoria in which your taste buds and brain are enticed. This experience is what keeps you coming back for more, hence the reason you may feel a loss of control once you dive into a bag of your favorite cookies, despite going in with the intention of having just one, or a couple, or five...you get the point.

Less Dancing, More Dieting

By choosing not to sign your taste buds up for daily dancing lessons, e.g., choosing to eat bland foods, you significantly increase the likelihood that you'll be able to stay strong on your diet, which means you hit your daily calorie goals and maximize progress.

Do you have to do this your entire diet? No. But myself, along with hundreds of clients in the past, have found this strategy successful when employed during the final 4-6 weeks of a diet (**when cravings are the worst**). Here's what you need to do to crush those cravings and salvage your diet:

1. **Choose Bland Foods**- Unfortunately, peanut butter is not a bland food. Neither is an egg (yolk included) omelet, or a well-marinated steak. However, raw vegetables, unflavored oats, egg whites, and plain Greek yogurt are bland.
Like, really bland.

What they provide in terms of health benefits, I think most of us will agree they lack in taste on their own.

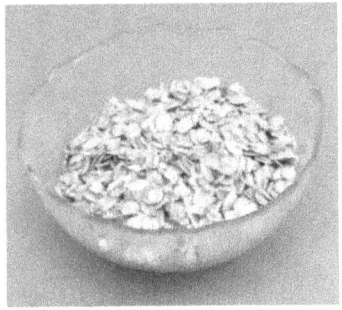 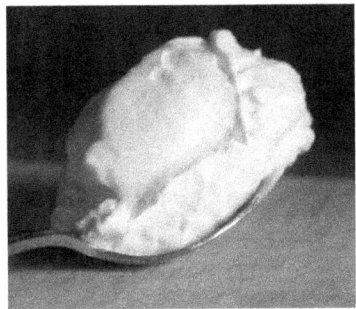

2. **Season Less**- Once you decide upon your staple bland foods, resist the urge to lather them with sauces, marinades, seasonings, and more. Stick with salt (it's essential) and nothing else.

   Keep it plain.
   Keep it boring.
   Keep it simple.

3. **Eat the Same Few Foods**- Numerous research studies show that you're more likely to overeat when faced with a variety of food options rather than the same food over and over.[5-7] So, yes, I am recommending you eat chicken, broccoli, and brown rice regularly, and **even more than once per day** during the final few weeks of a diet.

> *Put your variety on hold a few weeks and you'll be surprised*
> *how disinterested you become in food,*
> *which is advantageous at the tail end of a diet.*

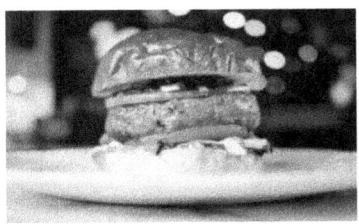

Consider a DIY burger made at home to save on calories (and money).

4. **Don't Dine Out**- Restaurants and chefs spend countless hours trying to increase the palatability of their foods to keep you coming back for more. This goes against everything we just discussed if you're looking to adhere to your diet. Put a pause on dining out for a few weeks. Your abs and wallet will thank you.

Chapter 5 Recap:

- Delicious food triggers a similar chemical response in your brain that drug addicts experience when using.

- Removing this euphoric feeling by eating bland food, especially towards the tail-end of a dieting phase when hunger and cravings are the strongest, may help you to finish your diet 100 percent on track.

- Consider choosing the same bland foods repeatedly throughout the day the final few weeks of your diet. Have a light hand on seasonings and sauces, too, to further keep food from becoming too flavorful.

- This approach is no forever – it's a strategy to use the final few weeks of a diet, or when cravings are beginning to become too strong.

CHAPTER 6: PRACTICE PORTION CONTROL

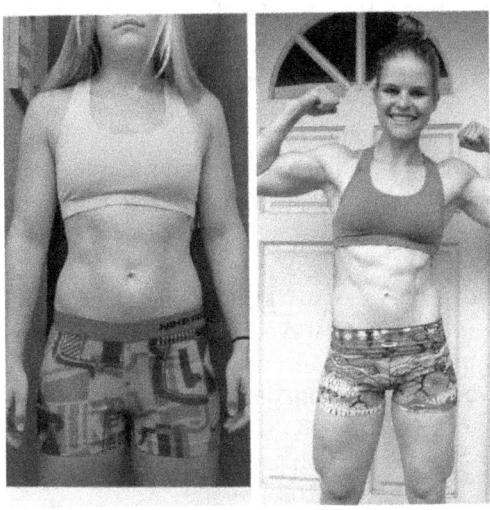

Raegan lost 7 pounds in 12 weeks!

It's 6:45 p.m. on a Monday and you've finally walked in the door after a long day of work. You know, the type of day filled with pointless meetings that led to absolutely nothing being accomplished, which means there will ultimately be even more meetings...

Yeah, one of those days.

As you walk inside you find that your new pup has left you a present in the kitchen. And the living room.

By the time you finally clean up each mess your pup left you, it's nearly 7:30 p.m.

You're starving.

You haven't eaten since lunch because of, well, meetings. At this point, your eyes are bigger than your stomach. And even despite your best eye-balling efforts, the fact that your brain is screaming "I'm starving!" cannot be ignored.

The result: you wind up piling on more food to your plate than you're supposed to have, or need. And if the portion of food happens to be a mighty calorie-dense dish, such as pasta, well, even the slightest oversight on portion control can have a major impact on your total calories for the day.

Size does matter.

If you're not **practicing portion control**, you're in for a lot of frustration during your diet. **Practice portion control** to ensure you are indeed taking in fewer calories than you're burning. Remember, that's essential for fat-loss.

You can eat clean, organic, gluten-free, and all of the above, but if you're not adhering to weight loss rule numero uno, it's for nothing. Yes, that's me telling you that it's possible to gain weight eating organic chicken and kale salads all day.

In the example above, there are two solutions that could significantly lower the risk of this portion misstep. First, you could have used a more reliable, and precise form of portion control. Secondly, you could have had a pre-portioned meal waiting for you at home. More on this later.

We will begin with the first solution.

Portion Control Strategies

Myself, as well as the hundreds of people I've worked 1:1 with, have the most success when utilizing a food scale to consistently and accurately **practice portion control**.

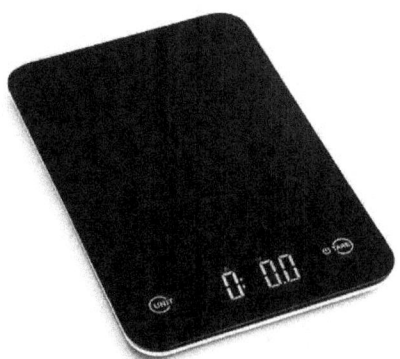

A food scale is invaluable if you're trying to lose weight. You should get one.

There's no better way to manage portions with precision. Unfortunately, the food scale is accompanied by a negative stigma. For the life of me, I cannot figure out why. It's as if you get the "oh you're one of those..." *look* when you mention having one, or guests see it in your kitchen.

Regardless of what others think, **it's an invaluable tool**. It will keep you honest and consistent.

Is There Another Way?

I'm a fan of mindful eating, "listening to your body," and even getting handsy with food to best delegate portions. But the major problem I find with these strategies, especially if you're new to dieting, or have struggled in the past, is that they can easily be overpowered by hunger and emotion. For some reason, despite aiming for a fistful of carbohydrates, I tend to end up with much more when I am hungry during a diet. Had I just measured out 200 grams (total weight) instead, I could have been done with it.

Can you relate?

Furthermore, these strategies can create additional decisions and ample opportunity to second guess yourself. A clear-cut portion as measured by a reliable scale takes the guesswork and anxiety out of the process. Two-hundred grams is 200 grams and there's no need or reason to rethink whether you need a bit more rice to make a fist-sized portion.

You need to put your food into a bowl or onto a plate anyway—what's the difference if there's a scale underneath?

Let Me Scale it Back

Utilizing a food scale isn't for everyone.

I get it.

To be honest, thousands of people have lost weight successfully without using a food scale. But if you're reading this book, I'd wager a guess that you've had some mixed results with past diets. If you want to finally earn the body you feel you've worked so hard for, this is the strategy I recommend to optimize your results.

I'm Out of Batteries...

When you're without a scale, or the scale batteries die (that's what they all say...) it's helpful to be familiar with a multitude of common portion sizes so you can best adapt to meet your meal nutrient needs.

Protein

Amount	Portion	
25 grams	1 palmful	
25 grams	1 scoop	

Carbohydrates

Amount	Portion	
50 grams	1¼ c cooked rice/pasta	
50 grams	1 c uncooked oats	
40 grams	1 c cooked rice/pasta/oats	
25 grams	1 medium fruit (tennis ball)	
15 grams	1 cup berries	

Fat

Amount	Portion	
15 grams	½ medium avocado	
15 grams	2 tbsp. nut butter	
15 grams	1 tbsp. oil	
15 grams	½ palm of nuts/seeds	

I'll Leave You with a Laugh

During preparation for my very first bodybuilding show, my food intake was pushed extremely low. So low that my only source of fat for the day was a ½-ounce of almonds with lunch and a tablespoon of peanut butter each night.

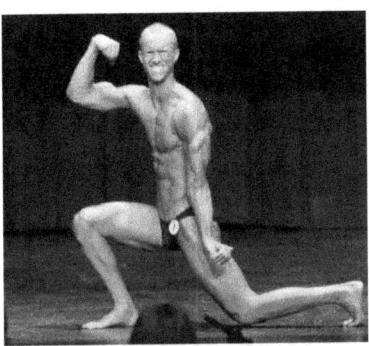

NGA Annapolis Cup, 2012: 1st place in the Novice Lightweight Division at a whopping 153 pounds!

I had weighed out every morsel of food and even measured out my condiments so that I would keep within my macronutrient guidelines for the day. For some reason, however, I never weighed out my peanut butter...

To this day, I am not sure why.

Well, after my competition, I decided to see just how much peanut butter I was consuming. I knew I was eating more than I was *supposedto*, but I was curious just how much more. My self-made meal plan called for 16 grams (7.5 grams of fat) of peanut butter with my bedtime meal. At the point of doing this test, I was a few weeks' post-competition. My food intake was up and I was no longer ravenous.

As you can imagine, before spooning that scoop of peanut butter, which I felt replicated my contest preparation habits, into my bowl, I undercompensated, thinking to myself, "there's no way I ate **that much**" as I put some back into the jar before transferring my spoonful to a bowl.
Well, despite reducing from my first replication attempt, the scale read: "48 grams."

Three times the amount I was *supposedto* have!

An additional 200 calories per day—which was very significant the final few weeks of prep!

So yeah, you could say I would've benefited from a bit of portion control with my calorie dense peanut butter.

The Bottom Line

If you want to optimize fat-loss, you need to **practice portion control**. The more outside noise you can remove from influencing your portions, e.g., hunger, and emotion, the more likely you are to stick to the proper amount of food you need to succeed during your fat-loss phase.

The approach I recommend: using a food scale as often as possible.

Chapter 6 Recap

- Portion control is vital when weight loss is your goal. It helps to ensure you're following the golden rule of weight loss: eat fewer calories than you're burning.

- A food scale is invaluable to ensure portion precision during a diet. It eliminates any second guessing and overpowers many emotional responses to food when both fatigue and hunger are high.

- Being familiar with common servings sizes of popular proteins, carbohydrates, and fats will be advantageous when using a food scale is not possible. Again, use of a food scale is highly encouraged to optimize diet progress.

CHAPTER 7: EAT EVERY THREE TO FIVE HOURS

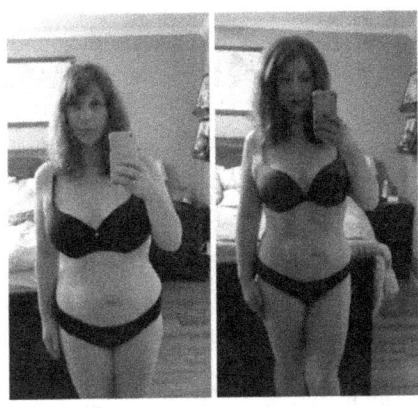

Marie lost 17 pounds in 13 weeks!

You can lose weight eating once per day. You can lose weight eating ten times per day.

What matters most is the relationship between the number of calories you eat and the number you burn each day.

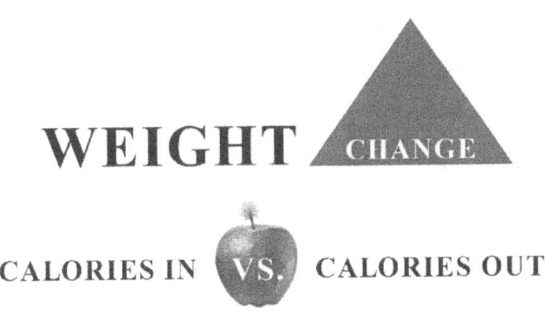

The golden rule of weight change.

However, in my years of helping hundreds of clients successfully lose fat (and keep it off!), I have found that eating every three to five hours is the approach that has had the most success.

Why?

Reason #1: To Optimize Muscle Growth and Repair

Throughout the day, your body is constantly building and breaking down new proteins. This is referred to as protein turnover. When you eat protein-rich foods, there's an increase in creation of new proteins within the body, and decrease in protein breakdown, which yields a net positive protein balance (which is necessary for muscle growth and repair).

#Winning

After a protein-rich meal, this increase in protein building reaches its peak between 90 – 120 minutes, and then returns to baseline around three hours later.[1] When protein building returns to baseline, your net protein balance becomes negative, meaning that you're breaking down more protein than you're building.

No Bueno.

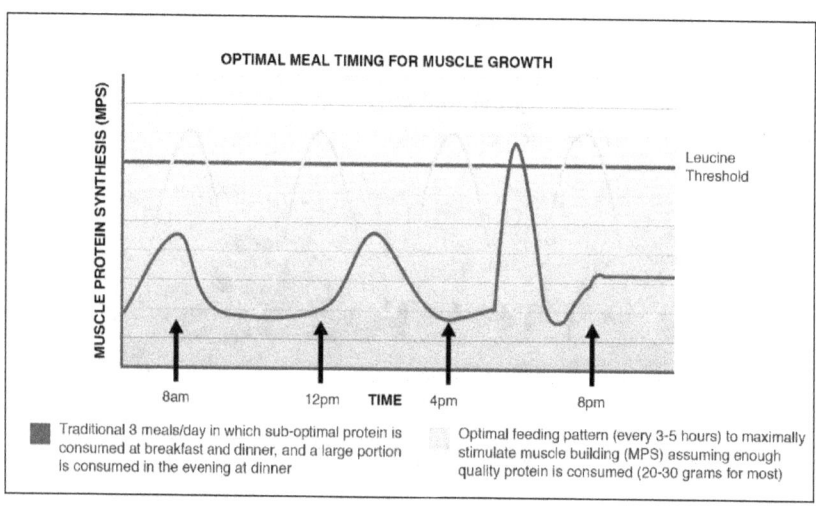

Eat every 3 – 5 hours to maximize muscle repair and growth.

At first glance, you may think that it makes sense to eat every 90 – 120 minutes. Unfortunately, your muscle machinery essentially becomes *numb* to a constant supply of protein, and there's no further elevation, or extension, in protein building when protein is constantly present.[2]

Translation: eating more frequently has no further benefit. If only...

But, **by eating every 3 – 5 hours**, you're able to optimize the amount of net-positive time throughout the day. This is crucial not only for suppressing hunger—see chapter one—but maximizing muscle maintenance, too. And since having more muscle helps to maintain the necessary calorie deficit needed to promote fat loss, this is highly desirable to drive fat loss without drastically cutting calories.

Reason #2: To Keep You Energized and Full

Your energy levels and appetite are tightly tied to your blood glucose levels.

A dip below your normal range (80 – 120 mg/dL for healthy persons) usually leads to fatigue, lightheadedness, dizziness, an inability to focus, and hunger.

Insulin is the hormone responsible for maintaining normal blood glucose levels. Following a meal, especially one rich in carbohydrates, blood glucose levels rise. How quickly they rise, and to what extent, are impacted by the type of food you eat and the size of your meal.

The spike in blood glucose triggers a release of insulin, which shuttles glucose in the blood for storage in either the liver or muscle tissue to reduce blood glucose levels back into a normal range. In healthy persons, blood glucose levels tend to be under 100 within two hours of finishing a meal.[3,4]*

For our purposes, I am discussing healthy persons, and not considering blood glucose and insulin impairment in pre-diabetic and diabetic populations.

As you spend a longer time between meals, blood glucose levels gradually decrease. That's because glucose is the primary fuel source for the brain, heart, central nervous system, and muscles. As you can imagine, the longer you go without food, the lower your blood glucose levels drop, which ultimately brings about some of the unwanted consequences I mentioned above.

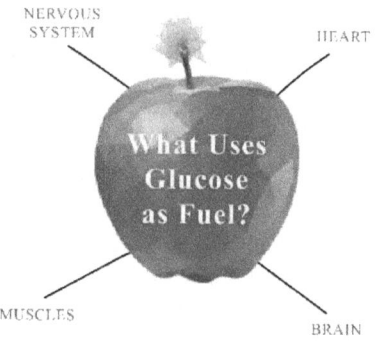

NERVOUS SYSTEM

HEART

What Uses Glucose as Fuel?

MUSCLES

BRAIN

Glucose serves as the primary fuel source for your brain, heart, muscles, and nervous system

By **eating every 3 – 5 hours**, you'll be able to maintain steady focus and energy, and able to keep hunger in check.

Reason #3: Flexibility and Individuality

Eating every three hours can be tough. Eating every – insert your favorite number here – is tough. That's because your schedule is not the same each day, no matter how badly you want it to be, and how hard you try to adjust. By giving yourself a range of time between meals, rather than a rigid number of hours, you'll be able to be flexible, and not stress about eating a meal 30 minutes later than you were *supposed* to.

Additionally, just because your coach, friend, or neighbor eats every three hours, doesn't mean that's optimal for you. You may find it best to strive for every four hours, yet some days it may be three and others five. Nonetheless, it fits to YOU.

What if I Can't Eat for Longer than Five Hours?

Eat when you can.

Seriously, don't stress about having to eat earlier or later than planned. It's going to happen. There will be times that you plan to eat a meal at 3:00 p.m., but get pulled into a meeting and end up not being able to eat until 6:00 p.m.

What you can do, however, is control whether you're prepared for such a situation, by having a convenient stash of healthy snacks available—at your desk, in your gym bag or purse, and at home. Convenient, travel-friendly snacks include: whey and casein protein, protein bars, protein chips, beef jerky, lean deli meat, low-fat Greek yogurt, oats, fruit, nuts, seeds, nut butters.

At the end of the day, do your best to still reach your calorie and macronutrient goals and move on to the next day.

Hunger Between Meals: A Friendly Reminder

Feeling hungry between meals while dieting is inevitable. Fortunately, after reading this book, you'll be armed with a multitude of strategies to crush hunger and minimize its appearance.

As a refresher, some of the strategies you can employ include the following:

1. **Prioritize Protein at Each Meal**- Remember, protein slows down digestion and directly influences appetite hormones to send satiety (fullness) signals to your brain.
2. **Choose High-Fiber Carbohydrates**- Fiber slows down digestion, ultimately taking up a lot of space in your stomach. This combination stretches the stomach, which sends satiety signals to your brain.
3. **Hydrate, Hydrate, Hydrate**- Fluids (quickly) take up a lot of space in your stomach, which promotes fullness. By drinking a lot of fluid before, during, after, and in between meals, you can strongly suppress hunger.
4. **Eat Vegetables at Every Meal**- Re-read fiber and hydration above ☺.

My Extended Hunger-Fighting Secret

If you know in advance, regardless of the reason, you'll have to go longer than five hours without a meal, consider making casein protein a part of your last meal before the gap.

Why?

Casein is a very slow to digest protein. This is because it clumps in the stomach. Thus, it provides a slow and steady release of amino acids to the muscles over the next 6 – 8 hours. This helps to keep you feeling full due to it occupying space in your stomach for the hours to come.

I personally like to take a scoop of whey protein, a scoop of casein protein, and a serving (or five) of peanut butter, and make a large bowl of protein pudding when I know I will be going a long period without food (such as before bed!).

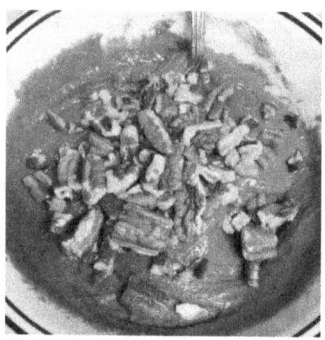

Get this tasty recipe and video in my YouTube channel.

Note: Dairy products are comprised of 80 percent casein and 20 percent whey. Low-fat Greek yogurt, cottage cheese, and milk are three excellent casein alternatives.

Chapter 7 Recap:

- Eating every 3 – 5 hours optimizes the positive impact a protein-rich food has on muscle growth and repair.

- Eating every 3 – 5 hours has a positive impact on blood glucose and energy levels, as well as your appetite.

- Eating every 3 – 5 hours promotes great flexibility and allows you to adapt your nutrition to your day as it constantly changes.

- If you need to go longer than five hours without food, consider using casein (or dairy) to provide your body with slow-digesting nutrients for the many hours to come.

CHAPTER 8: COOK, PREPARE,
AND PACK FOOD IN BULK (AND IN ADVANCE)

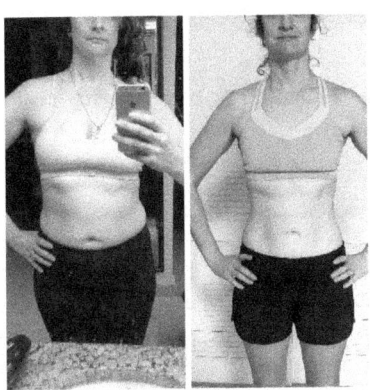

Charlotte lost 13 pounds in 13 weeks during our first diet together. She then lost
another 16 pounds in 12 weeks (the second diet began roughly 18 weeks after her first one)!

Earlier, we learned first-hand the impact a long, stressful day at work can have on your ability to rationally portion foods. At the end of the day, both physical and emotional factors are in play. You are not only physically hungry—remember the pointless meetings you got stuck in that led to missing a meal—but you're also in dire need of a pick-me-up.

And what better source of happiness than tasty food? Especially, in large amounts!

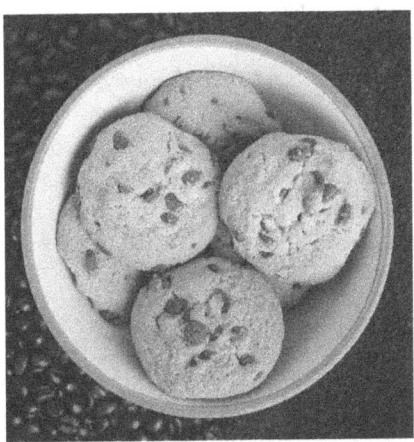

Cookies and other treats can be the downfall of your diet
when you don't have meals prepared and hunger gets the best of you.

But as I briefly eluded to, and promised we'd return to…

…aside from utilizing a food scale to keep you on track, I strongly recommend you **cook, prepare, and pack food in bulk (and in advance)**. What you save in the days to come is invaluable and worth every second of what you invest up front.

Prepping Per Meal Versus Prepping in Bulk

I'll be candid; **cooking, preparing, and packing food in bulk (and in advance)** takes time…at first.

However, there are innumerable strategies you can employ to **cut this time in half** and streamline the process. More on this in a bit. What I want to first focus on is the tremendous savings you reap when deciding to tackle a large meal prep endeavor rather than a "one meal at a time" approach.

For starters, you save a lot of time. If you take the "one meal at a time" approach, you must factor in the following time commitment **each** time you eat:

1. **Preparation**- Any slicing, dicing, marinating that is required may take 5 – 15 minutes.
2. **Cooking**- Depending on what you're cooking, and what method(s) you're using, this may range from 2 – 60 minutes.
3. **Cooling**- Unless you have an iron tongue, the food you cook needs to cool for at least 10 – 15 minutes.

The entire meal process, from start to finish, may cost you 60 minutes (or more!) of time. **And this is just for one meal!** Of course, you could always rely on frozen meals, or fast-food…but, I think there's a better approach.

By preparing food in bulk, you can simultaneously cook food for multiple meals, while saving a fortune of time over the long-run. Sure, total prep time may increase by 10 – 15 minutes, but the time to cook food (depending on cooking method) shouldn't significantly change (your baking pan can hold more than one chicken breast and your oven more than one pan), and cooling time will remain relatively unaffected, too.

Choosing to cook in bulk takes care of 95 percent of the prep-cook-eat process at once. All that's left is to reheat the food whenever you want to enjoy it, and this takes only a few minutes. And during those few minutes, you can catch up on one my latest articles,nutrition nuggets, or, even learn everything you need to know about your favorite nutrients.

...seriously, you should open a few articles or videos in a separate tab to read or watch later.

Decision Making

Making decisions can be stressful. This is especially true for decisions related to food when you're fatigued, irritated, and haven't eaten in a while. The chances are, that when you're in this state, you're more apt to choose a convenient, high-calorie food, rather than taking the time to prepare a healthy meal to support your fat-loss goals.

By **cooking, preparing, and packing food in bulk (and in advance)**, you'll now be able to come home to an already pre-thought out, pre-portioned, pre-cooked meal that requires just a few minutes to be ready to eat. Oh, and did I mention this strategy can apply to your breakfast, lunch, dinner, and snacks? No longer do you need to rely on office donuts, or lunch time fast-food trips for your meals. You can prep any meal or snack in bulk and in advance!

Note: A Word on Will Power

Each time you make a decision,you flex your willpower muscle and fatigue it.

Just like any other muscle in your body, this muscle fatigues as you use it more and more. Your will power is a muscle that you flex innumerable times throughout the day. Think what to wear, what to eat, what to email, what to text, what to comment on social media...you get the point.

By creating specific habits, or eliminating decision-making occasions by preparing in advance, you help to save willpower.At the end of the work day you've used quite a bit of willpower. Why do you think it's a struggle for so many to go to the gym after work? They're drained. Not just physically, but mentally, and emotionally, too.

By **cooking, preparing, and packing food in bulk (and in advance)**, you create a situation in which you don't have to think about what or how much to eat. You don't need to tap into that willpower muscle to portion out or cook your next meal. Instead, you can virtually operate on autopilot and stay on track with your fat-loss efforts.

Make Meal Prep Efficient

For many, the act or thought of meal prepis akin to spending the day with that distant relative who doesn't stop talking and always says whatever is on his or her mind.

Both sound dreadful.

But meal prep doesn't have to be like that.

In fact, it can be done much quicker than you think and can even be enjoyable—put on some tunes, a podcast, a Nutrition Nugget, or your favorite TV show and get to it!

Before you do get your hands dirty, there are a few key steps that must be taken to make your meal prep efficient.

1. **Decide on a Day(s)-** Select a day (or two) that you will be **cooking, preparing, and packing food in bulk (and in advance)**. Many find that they have the most time on a Saturday or Sunday, while others prefer to do it on a Tuesday. There's no right or wrong approach—find the day(s) that works best for you.

    If you decide to spread meal prep across more than one day, you need to decide which meals will be prepared. Will you prepare food on Sunday for Monday through Wednesday and then prepare food Wednesday evening for Thursday through Saturday? Or, will you prepare food on Sunday for Monday through Saturday? Again, there's no wrong approach—find what works for you.

2. **Narrow Down Number of Meals-** Which meals will you be prepping for the week? Lunch for every day? Lunch and dinner for Monday through Wednesday? Whether it's five meals, or ten, you need to know ahead of time so that you can purchase the appropriate amount of food and allocate enough time.

    Decide What You Will Eat- What will you eat at each meal? Will it be the same food each meal, each day of the week? There's research to support this habit for fighting hunger and cravings while on a diet. Review chapter five or click here to learn more. Whether it's a Tupperware of overnight oats in the morning and salmon and greens in the afternoon, knowing in advance will enable you to streamline shopping, purchasing, and preparing.

I recommend that you keep a few staple items for both lean proteins and healthy carbohydrates and rotate between them throughout the weeks. For instance, my go-to protein sources for lunch are salmon, ground turkey, and roasted chicken. My go-to carbohydrate sources are brown rice and sweet potatoes. I find each of these simple to **cook, prepare, and pack food in bulk (and in advance)**, and I still leave myself with the option of alternating tastes and combinations as I wish.

3. **Pick Your Portions Per Meal**- If you don't know your portions per meal ahead of time, it will be a struggle buying the appropriate amount of food for the week. There's nothing worse than beginning meal prep only to find yourself 12 ounces short on flank steak, and 2 cups short on quinoa (okay, there's plenty worse, but it's still less than ideal).
    If you plan to have 4-ounces of flank steak five times per week, you need a total of 20-ounces for the week. **HOWEVER**, you need to keep in mind that most meats lose roughly 25 percent of their total weight during cooking. Therefore, you'll need to buy 25-ounces of flank steak to ensure you have 20-ounces cooked (20 multiplied by 1.25 equals 25). Click HERE to learn more about how cooking impacts your protein.

Once you have a plan, the food you need, and the appropriate portions, it's time to dive in! To minimize time spent in the kitchen, it's important that you devise an optimal flow to enable foods to cook simultaneously, while also affording you the opportunity to tend to the food that doesn't need to be cooked.

Time Saving Equipment

If you don't already have these pieces of kitchen equipment, I highly encourage that you invest in them. They're quite affordable.

1. **Crock Pot**- Rather than tending to the veggies you're sautéing, the chicken you're searing, and constantly eyeing the pasta that's borderline bubbling over all at once, using a crock pot allows you to take a "prepare and forget" approach.

   In less than 15 minutes, you can add your favorite lean protein, healthy carbohydrate, and vegetable to one big pot, and hit start. Then, you can go about your day for the next 4 – 8 hours and come back to a deliciously smelling, perfectly cooked batch of food. The best part is that if you buy a large enough crock pot, this meal can serve as dinner tonight and each night of the week. Talk about a time saving, efficient way to prep your meals!

2. **Rice Cooker**- Add rice. Add water. Press "cook." That's all it takes to initiate the cooking process. Within 45 – 60 minutes, you'll have fluffy, perfectly cooked rice. And during that time, you can knock out all other meal prep needs instead of constantly stressing about whether you added enough water and if the water is going to boil over.

3. **George Forman Grill**- It's very cost friendly and is another efficient way to prepare your food. It's a time saver when you compare the minutes it takes to prep, light, and start a regular grill (depending on what you have), and it provides a similar cook time compared to pan-roasting your lean protein, or baking it in the oven.

   The major advantage it holds over previously mentioned methods, however, is it's a quick cooking method, which provides you grill-like taste in a short amount of time. And let's not kid ourselves—everything tastes better grilled!

Bulk Food Prep Staples

Below is a list of food items that I have found to help further enhance my meal prep efficiency:
1. Frozen vegetables
2. Bulk-cooked proteins
3. Bulk-cooked rice and pasta
4. Overnight Oats
5. Hard-Boiled Eggs

A Day in the Life Of

Below I have outlined an in-depth look into my weekly meal prep routine for the purpose of showing you how I maximize every second of the process to get it done in as little time as possible.

When: Sunday

Time: 60 – 70 minutes

Outcome: 2 meals/day Monday – Friday; 10 meals total.

Meal #1: Pork tenderloin, brown rice, frozen vegetables

Meal #2: A salad paired with roasted chicken and a side of blueberry overnight oats

Complete Meal Plan Steps:

1. Preheat the oven to 350 degrees Fahrenheit.
2. I line a baking dish with foil and place chicken in dish and season both sides. Wash hands.
3. Add three cups of rice and six cups of water to rice cooker and start the cooking process.
4. Once the oven is preheated, place chicken in oven and set timer (24- 27 minutes).
5. Dice three bell peppers into slim strips. Then, add a handful of spring mix, a handful of carrots, and a handful of bell pepper slices to a Tupperware container. Add portions so people know how much you use (like what you did for the oats)

Next, I begin on the overnight oats: Five containers of overnight oats: 1 cup oats, ½ cup Greek yogurt, ½ cup fruit, cinnamon to taste.

1. I add oats to every Tupperware, followed by Greek yogurt, and cinnamon.
2. Then, I add water (enough to for all ingredients to soak up and form a viscous consistency, about ½-cup) to each Tupperware, stir, and then repeat for each.
3. I then top with blueberries and place in refrigerator.

Then, I shift focus to preparing my pork meal. Remember, the chicken and rice are both still in the oven at this point.

1. I add 1 – 2 handfuls of frozen vegetables to five empty Tupperware containers. Seal and place them in the fridge.
2. By this time, the chicken is done or nearly done. Once the chicken is finished, I take it out of the oven, and let it cool for 10 minutes. I then turn the oven up to 415 degrees Fahrenheit.
3. Next, I add new foil to the baking dish, and take out a stovetop pan, and set a burner to high heat.
4. I season my pork tenderloin (only the top) and begin searing the pork (seasoning the bottom once I've placed the piece face down on the pan). I sear the pork for 60 – 90 seconds on each side, before transferring to the baking dish. Then, I finish it in the over for an additional 10 – 12 minutes.
5. Once the pork is in the oven, I begin slicing the chicken and portioning into Ziploc bags (this will go with my salad).
6. Once my pork tenderloin is finished, I take out of the oven and let stand for 10 minutes. I then slice, portion, and add it to the previously prepared Tupperware containers of frozen vegetables.
7. Now, I may be waiting on the rice for another 10 – 15 minutes (depending on how much I make). I put everything away in the fridge and let the rice cool for 15- 20 minutes.
8. I begin cleaning at this point.
9. Once it's had time to cool, I portion out the appropriate amount into the Tupperware containers with pork and frozen veggies—this takes another three minutes.
10. I soak the pot I cooked the rice in and boom: 15 meals in roughly 60 minutes!

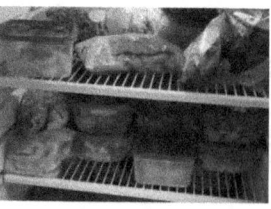

10 meals prepared in 60 minutes!

Chapter 8 Recap:

- Cooking, preparing, and packing food in bulk (and in advance) can save you hours of time in the kitchen throughout the week.

- To maximize the efficiency of your meal prep, it's important that you have a plan and know the following information:
    - How many days per week you'll be preparing food.
    - Which days and how many meals need to be prepared.
    - What food you will be preparing for each meal.
    - What portions of each food item you will need.

- Consider investing in time-saving kitchen equipment such as a crockpot, rice cooked, or George Forman grill.

- Learn to multi-task to enhance efficiency.

CHAPTER 9: EAT MORE FOOD LATER IN THE DAY

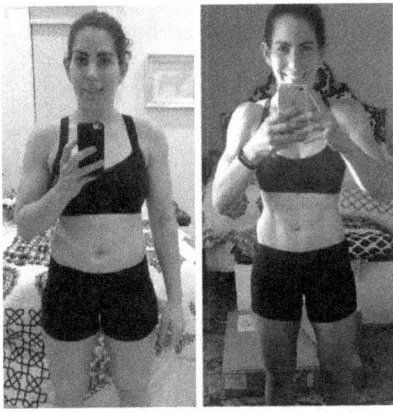

Alissa lost 14 pounds in 13 weeks!

Think about the last time you had a cheat meal...

Was it 9:30 a.m. in the office, or 9:30 p.m. on your couch in front of the TV?

If I had to wager a bet, I'd guess the latter.

There are many factors in play as to why hunger and cravings hit hardest in the evening, which I will explain in further detail shortly. Therefore, I recommend **you eat more food later in the day**. Of course, it's still essential that you're eating the appropriate amount to stay in the necessary deficit to drive fat loss because eating more than your needs, well, that can wreak havoc on your goals.

A Typical Day...

Your alarm goes off at 6:00 a.m.

You take a shower, brush your teeth, and head out the door (hopefully) with a few meals or snacks to carry you throughout the day.

After 30 minutes of driving and listening to your favorite pump-up music, podcast, or talk radio, you arrive at work ready to tackle the day.

As you settle at your desk, you begin checking Facebook and the local news. Before diving into the first task of the day, you prepare yourself a cup of delicious tasting office coffee. You take a deep breath, check your Instagram one last time, and then it's off to the races...

Before you know it, it's nearly 12:00 p.m., which means time for lunch. After an hour-long lunch break chit chatting with friends, texting with your significant other, and watching a TNT University course video, you turn your attention to preparing for a couple of afternoon meetings and finishing a presentation for later in the week.

Before you know it, it's nearly 5:00 p.m. and the work day is over.

Yet, all you've had so far is a protein shake for breakfast and a peanut butter sandwich for lunch...

By the time you get home, it's 6:00 p.m. and for the remainder of the evening you have nothing on your plate—literally. It's time for dinner, and, well, whatever else you choose to do.

This is when the night gets interesting, and diets are usually broken.

Why You're Not Hungry During the Day

You're not hungry during the day for a handful of reasons:

1. Appetite hormones are low in the morning, meaning you're not hungry immediately upon awakening.
2. Your morning coffee or tea works to suppress appetite.
3. Stress steadily climbs during the day, which suppresses appetite.
4. Your focus is OFF food, and on the day's tasks, meetings, and calls. Some days it may feel as if you don't have even a second to think about food.

As you can see, this combination can nip hunger in the bud quickly. But by the time you get home, you have an empty plate, metaphorically speaking, and a raging appetite.

Consequences of the Late-Night Binge

We've all had a night where we can't stop after one bite of ice cream, one cookie, or one spoonful of peanut butter...

Or even worse, a night composed of all three!

This behavior and lack of control may leave you with an additional 750 – 1,000 calories for the day. And although this is only one night—at least I hope so—it can have a major ripple effect on your progress for the next day, week, or even across the entire diet itself.

Here's how:

Let's assume you're in a daily deficit of 300 calories.

Well, after a few too many spoonfuls of peanut butter, you end up in a substantial calorie surplus—let's say 700-calorie surplus for this example (1,000 calories from peanut butter minus the 300 from your planned deficit nets a surplus of 700 calories). The first area this impact is felt is in at tomorrow's weigh-in.It should come to no surprise that tomorrow's weight will be higher than you'd like.*

*Note: Diet deviations happen to the best of us. If you happen to veer off plan, consider passing on the next day's weigh-in (if that happens to be your scheduled day). It will save you a lot of stress.

But in a bigger light, this night of deviation knocks your total weekly deficit of a planned 2,100 calories down to 1,400, which means the next few weigh-ins may be undesirable. This can take a major toll on your emotional state, especially if you live and die by the scale—don't worry, I will talk about strategies to break this habit in a later chapter. After 5 – 7 days of no progress (as evidenced by the scale), your frustration may reach an all-time high, and as a means of comforting yourself, you decide to hang out with Ben and Jerry, or your buddy Jiffy, once again.

And the vicious cycle begins again...

But by strategically setting up your nutrition to afford you more calories in the evening (with a higher-protein approach during the day compared to before), you'll be able to eat substantially more calories in the evening, which will leave you feeling plenty full before bed, yet within your daily calorie goal.

This will come as a nice change of pace if you're used to feeling ravenous after 5:00 p.m.

Strategies to Fight Nighttime Hunger and Cravings

As the name of the chapter suggests, I want you to **eat more food later in the day**, and to capitalize on the fact that you're not too hungry during the first part of the day. Here are a few strategies to use when setting up your daily nutrition:

1. **Shift Calories Later in the Day**- Rather than spreading your calories out evenly across the day, skew your distribution to include higher-calorie meals later in the evening.

   Calorie Distribution During the Day:

	Meal #1	Meal #2	Meal #3	Meal #4	Meal #5
Even Distribution	500	500	500	500	500
Skewed Distribution	250	250	500	750	750

2. **Eat More Protein Later in the Day**- You're aware of the hunger-suppressing benefits protein offers (for a refresher, review chapter one). By eating more protein in the evening, you'll significantly slow digestion and trigger a cascade of hormone release that serves to signal satiety. Add an ounce or two to each of your latter meals (meals 4 and 5 in this instance) to better promote fullness.

   Note: Protein should still be a focal point at each meal earlier in the day.

   Protein Distribution During the Day (ounces/meal):

	Meal #1	Meal #2	Meal #3	Meal #4	Meal #5
Even Distribution	4	4	4	4	4
Skewed Distribution	4	4	4	6	6

3. **Eat More Vegetables Later in the Day**- As you recall from chapter three, vegetables pack a beautiful blend of fiber and fluids that stop hunger in its tracks. You should be eating them at every meal. If you are someone who struggles with nighttime hunger, eating more vegetables at dinner and as a bedtime snack will help to promote fullness without adding many calories.

Vegetable Distribution During the Day (handful servings/meal):

	Meal #1	Meal #2	Meal #3	Meal #4	Meal #5
Even Distribution	1	1	1	1	1
Skewed Distribution	1	1	2	2 – 3	2 – 3

4. **Save Fats for the Evening-** Fat also slows digestion and can help promote fullness. Save at least half of your fat for the evening so that you can have a larger dinner and bedtime meal to keep hunger and cravings in check. This will afford you significantly more calories in the evening to eat.

Fat Distribution During the Day (percent of calories):

	Meal #1	Meal #2	Meal #3	Meal #4	Meal #5
Even Distribution	20	20	20	20	20
Skewed Distribution	10	15	15	30	30

Sample Day: P.M. Workout

Meal #	Meal Composition
1	Protein, veggies
2	Protein, fat, veggies
3	Protein, carbohydrates, veggies
4	Protein, carbohydrates, fats, veggies
5	Protein, carbohydrates, fats, veggies

What if I Exercise in the Morning?

You can still implement the above recommended strategies if you train in the morning. You still should be eating ample protein and vegetables at each meal, and should also focus on carbohydrates at both the pre- and post-workout meal.

If you're keen on *saving* carbohydrates for the evening, reduce the portion of carbohydrates you consume at the pre- and post-workout meal by 25 percent. Additionally, you can move almost all fat for the day to the later meals, which will do wonders for mental and physical satiety.

Sample Day: A.M. Workout

Meal #	Meal Composition
1	Protein, carbohydrates, veggies
2	Protein, carbohydrates, veggies
3	Protein carbohydrates, veggies
4	Protein, fats, veggies
5	Protein, fats, veggies

Chapter 9 Recap:

- Hunger is often absent early in the morning and throughout the day due to low levels of appetite hormones upon waking, appetite suppression from daily coffee or tea, business of work, and stress levels.

- Strategically placing a larger amount of your daily allotted calories to later in the day can help reduce the likelihood of binge-eating and eating off plan.

- Consider increasing the amount of protein and vegetables per meal in the evening.

- Move a majority of your carbohydrates and fats to the last two meals of your day; keep daily meals focused on protein and vegetables.

CHAPTER 10: AVOID ALCOHOL

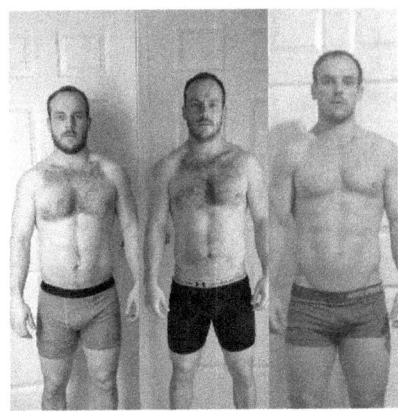

Luke lost 18 pounds in 12 weeks!

By now, you should realize that the underlying tone of this book is "optimization." I am providing you with recommendations to optimize your efforts and progress during a diet. If you can make subtle, consistent changes to your day, well, it could be the difference between seeing six abs versus two, getting eight muscle-ups versus four, or losing 16 pounds instead of 10 when all is said and done.

One of the easiest changes you can make to drive fat-loss is to **avoid alcohol**. This isn't a permanent change, but during the next 12 – 14 weeks, if you want to optimize progress, **avoid alcohol**.

The Obvious Reasons

Alcohol contains calories.

Seven calories per gram, to be exact, which is nearly twice as many per gram compared to protein and carbohydrates (each provide four calories per gram), and nearly as many as a gram of fat (which provides nine calories per gram).

It should be self-explanatory that drinking alcohol means you're consuming more calories. And given that one drink is typically well over 100 calories, your necessary calorie deficit to drive fat-loss is gone in a flash.

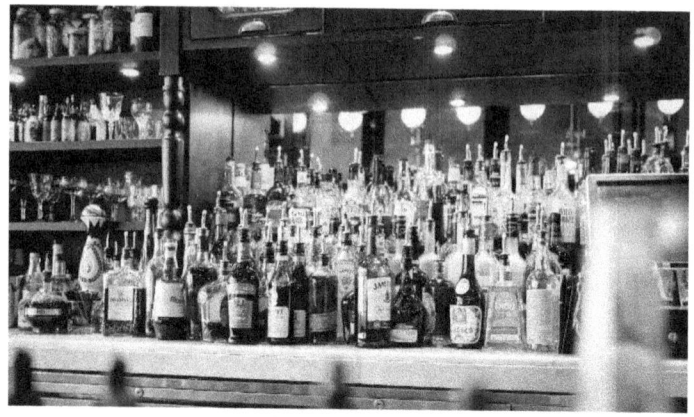

The impact alcohol has on fat loss goes beyond the calorie contribution...

As with most any decision in life, there's always some form of a ripple effect. In this case, not only does drinking alcohol add more calories to your day from the alcohol itself, but it's also typically accompanied by a loss of any rational decision making when it comes to choosing nutritious foods. This sets you up to consume a smorgasbord of high-calorie options.

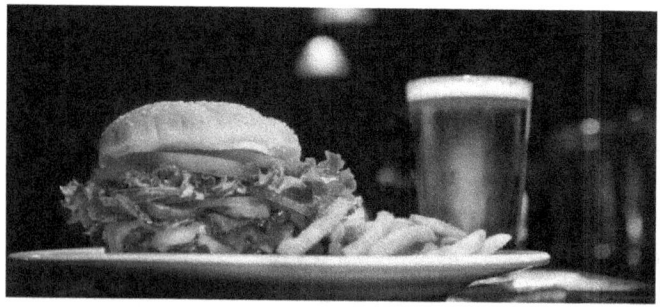

Regular burgers and beer isn't a part of your typical diet...

Think of your typical bar foods and favorite late-night munchies...

The last bar I went to didn't have happy hour pricing on veggie kabobs, salads, and fresh fruit. Rather, staple options included nachos, mozzarella sticks, burgers, fries, and practically anything deep fried, or covered in grease!

The common denominator of these foods is **that they're extremely calorie-dense**. Combine this with the calorie-laden alcohol and you very well may hit your daily calorie goal in one meal! Not an ideal approach for fat loss, to say the least.

A Shot of Science

Beyond the excess number of calories you're bound to consume when indulging in alcohol, there's a deeper, more significant change going on in your body that's further working against your fat-loss efforts.

Your body views alcohol as a toxin.

Once ingested, your body immediately shifts its resources and priorities to removing alcohol. Thus, other processes take the backseat and come to a screeching halt until alcohol is removed. Depending on your age, gender, size, and the amount you drink, this can last quite a few hours!

Once alcohol is consumed, your body immediately breaks it down into a molecule known as acetaldehyde. It's this very step that catalyzes an undesirable chain reaction. From here, acetaldehyde is further broken down into an intermediary molecule known as acetyl-coA.

$$\text{Alcohol} \rightarrow \text{acetaldehyde} + \text{NADH} \rightarrow \text{acetyl-coA} \rightarrow \text{fat storage}$$

Acetyl-CoA is an intermediate molecule for protein, carbohydrate, and fat metabolism. An excessive build-up of Acetyl-CoA can lead to increased formation of fatty acids, which eventually leads to **increased fat storage**.

Additionally, another byproduct of alcohol metabolism is increased production of a molecule known as nicotinamide adenine dinucleotide (NADH), which increases to facilitate alcohol breakdown. An increase in NADH is a signal that there's plenty of energy available (which is obvious given you just consumed calorie-containing alcohol). This increase in NADH further favors fatty acid formation, as well as energy storage.[1]

Again, not ideal for your fat-loss efforts.

Final Thoughts...

Some of you reading this may have been hopeful that I recommended moderation, or a specific type of alcohol to minimize the damage it inflicts on your fat-loss efforts.

Sorry, not sorry.

Let me remind you that one major reason you purchased this book is because you've struggled with previous diets, or feel that your efforts are not reflected in the mirror, in the gym, or on the scale.

If you want to get the most out of your hard work in the gym and kitchen and optimize progress, **avoid alcohol** during a diet.

Period.

It's not forever.

In the meantime, replace your usual alcoholic beverage with a crisp and refreshing carbonated beverage of choice. A diet soda on ice with a spritz of lime juice, now that's a treat.

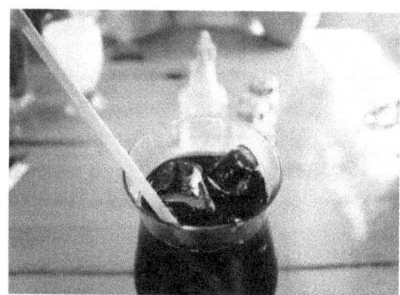

Mmmmm.... a virgin rum and coke.

Chapter 10 Recap:

- Avoiding alcohol during your diet can have a tremendous impact on your progress.

- Alcohol not only adds more calories to your day, but increases the likelihood of consuming high-calorie food, too.

- Alcohol is a toxin. Your body stops what it's doing to remove alcohol when you drink it. This means fat burning is put on pause. Simultaneously, fat storage is increased as your body views this overload of excess calories as an opportunity to store up to combat the present stress (your diet).

CHAPTER 11: DON'T RELY ON THE SCALE

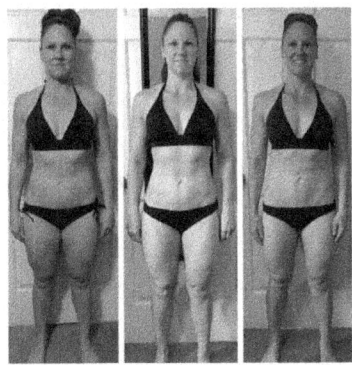

Brandie lost 11 pounds in 11 weeks during her first diet with me,
and then, 14 weeks later, she lost an additional 7 pounds over 10 weeks!

Consider the following two situations:
You just trudged through the twelfth week of your diet. Hurriedly, you make your way to the local donut shop following your final morning weigh-in.

To date, you've lost 18 pounds.

But throughout the past 12 weeks, despite the weight loss and your clothes fitting loosely, you've been miserable. Hunger has been constant, fatigue your new best friend, and you've taken a few steps backwards in the gym.

But hey, 18 pounds in 12 weeks, that's not too shabby. And for now, you're celebrating, by purchasing a dozen donuts for the office. Did I mention you work from home by yourself?

Or, consider the alternative scenario:

You've just stepped on the scale to record your final weigh-in, which culminates twelve weeks of dieting. The morning number indicates you've lost 8 pounds the past 12 weeks. Out of the corner of your eye, you catch a glance of your stomach in the mirror, and stop to admire newly visible muscle you didn't know existed.

Slowly, a large smile comes across your face...

Finally, you're proud of how you look.

You've leaned out in all the right places, it's time to buy smaller sizes in your clothes, and even more impressive, your performance has improved almost weekly since beginning the diet.

And although you're certainly looking forward to a larger than usual meal this evening, your hunger is manageable, and you're quite content waiting until this evening to celebrate 12 weeks of hard work. And you don't plan on any of the sound nutritional behaviors you've learned the past 12 weeks; you just plan to gradually increase food.

Hopefully, you'd prefer to go through the latter situation. Yes, in the former, you've lost 10 more pounds. But is feeling like crap for a majority of a diet and having a much higher likelihood of post-diet, rapid weight regain really worth a few extra digits on the scale?

I'll let you decide for yourself...

Don't rely on the scale to gauge your progress.

Doing so will hide the many other positive changes taking place, and ultimately place a negative cloud over your hard work.

Many Variables Impact Your Morning Weigh-In

You just weighed in at a new diet low. WOO!

Tomorrow, however, the scale tells a different story. You're up two pounds.

"How the heck did I gain two pounds of fat overnight?" you exclaim out loud. "I ate the same exact thing, and my workout was longer than usual!"

Does that sound familiar?

I bet it does.

And that's okay.

We've all been there.

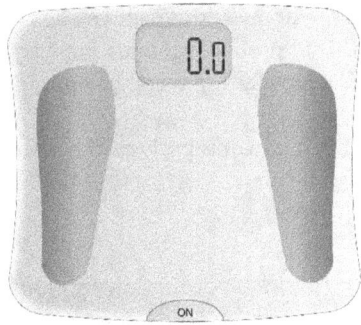

The scale is impacted by numerous variables – don't rely on it as the only indicator of progress.

Your body weight will fluctuate daily. This is because many variables impact your morning weigh-in, specifically, your previous day's food, fluids, and sodium intake. Yes, drinking an extra glass of water, or adding an extra couple pinches of salt to dinner, can influence the number on the scale.

Furthermore, your stress levels, sleep schedule, and change in hormones during the menstrual cycle, all impact your morning weigh-in, too. And if yesterday's workout was a doozie, the chances are you're sorer than usual, thus, have some significant inflammation going on, which translates to water retention and a higher number on the scale.

Take a deep breath.

Don't get caught up in one scale number as it is common to fluctuate a few pounds on any given day. Furthermore, recognize that weight loss is not linear. It often looks something like this:

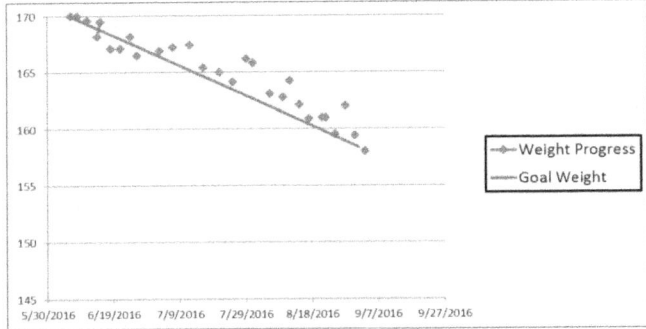

If you expect a new low weight each time you weigh in
you are setting yourself up for failure from the beginning.

One day you're down three pounds, the next you're up two, and the following you're down one again. That probably sounds familiar. But that day you're up two pounds...my guess is it's by far the worst day of the week.

That's why it's important that **you don't rely on the scale** to gauge your progress.

The Progress Puzzle

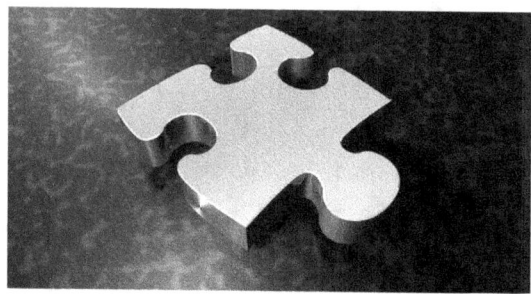

The scale is just one piece of the progress puzzle.

Fortunately, this isn't a two- or three-piece puzzle set. There are numerous other indicators of progress that you need to consider.

- Increase in energy
- Increase in workout performance
- Increase in workout recovery
- Increase in nutrition knowledge
- Increase in confidence
- Positive change in body composition
- Clothes fit loosely
- Decrease in stress levels

And in my opinion, these changes are **far more valuable** than a number on the scale. If you invest too much time and energy into the scale, it'll dominate your day; thus, you'll become increasingly frustrated with your *lack of progress* (despite many other positive changes taking place!) and potentially stray from your plan. And of course, you're aware at this point the ripple effect that can follow an emotional binge or break from your diet.

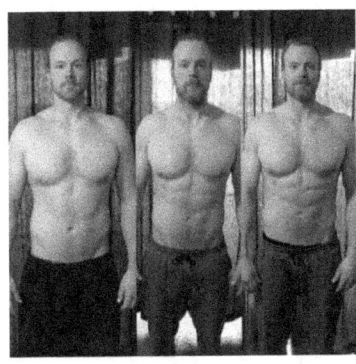

Progress photos tell a better story of progress compared to the scale.

Instead, acknowledge the scale for what it is—a piece of the progress puzzle, or one of many tools to assess progress—and appreciate the big picture, and several other changes taking place.

How Often Should I Weigh Myself?

There are two major schools of thought regarding optimal weigh-in frequency for weight loss.

On one end, there are those who believe in the once per week approach. A major pro of this approach is that it takes a lot of stress and anxiety out of the equation because one doesn't have to face the scale too often.

On the other hand, because your weight may fluctuate a few pounds daily, weekly weigh-ins may not accurately portray what progress is truly occurring. What if you had a very salty snack the day before your once weekly weigh-in?

Furthermore, a study out of Psychological Reports found that weekly weigh-ins, the method of choice for many popular group weight-loss meetings, motivated many people to "beat the scale" by engaging in unhealthy weight-control practices in an effort not to look bad or feel embarrassed.[1]

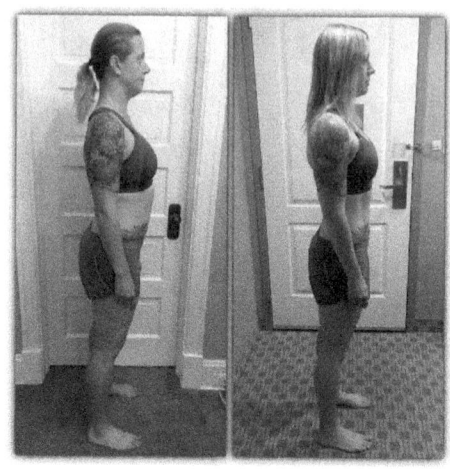

Weighing in once per week may not be enough to paint an accurate picture of progress.

On the opposite side, there exists the daily weigh-in camp. This approach provides multiple data points to quickly discern a true trend in weight change. It may also help to encourage accountability and provide you the opportunity to quickly realize when you've gone too far off track. Conversely, it also can lead to becoming overly dependent on the scale, which has the potential to lead to many unhealthy, and potentially, disordered behaviors.

The Sweet Spot: I recommend choosing 2 – 3 days per week. Either Monday and Thursday, or, Monday, Wednesday, Friday has worked well for the hundreds of individuals I have worked with that <u>successfully lost weight (and kept it off)</u>.

Rate of Weight Loss

Your weight loss efforts should lead to a loss of 0.5 – 1.0 percent of your body weight per week. This amounts to 0.75 – 1.5 pounds per week for a 150-pound person, or 1.0 – 2.0 pounds per week for a 200-pound person.

To best assess your progress—from the scale point of view, which, again, is only one piece of the progress puzzle—plan to weigh yourself two or three days per week. When doing so, make sure you weigh yourself right upon waking after using the restroom.

Next, find the average of those days and then proceed to compare to the previous week's average. If you're within the 0.5 – 1.0 percent weight loss sweet spot, there's no need to change anything. If your weight change more closely resembles a flat line, then it may be time to go back to the drawing board and consider tweaking calories and macros, or adjusting your exercise routine.

However, if you feel great, hold steady another week – what's the rush?

If you're losing weight faster than this recommended rate, especially in back-to-back weeks, that's a sign you should put a break on weight loss and add a bit more food back in. **Losing weight too quickly can lead to significant muscle loss and unnecessary levels of hunger.**

Both are no Bueno.

Chapter 11 Recap:

- Many variables impact the number on the scale, including: previous day's food, fluid, and sodium intake, stress levels, sleep, hormones, timing in the menstrual cycle, and past exercise.

- The scale is just one piece of the progress puzzle. Many other indicators of progress should be considered during a diet to truly assess the plan to date. Examples include: change in energy, exercise performance, body composition, confidence, nutrition knowledge, and well-being.

- A healthy rate of weight loss is 0.5 – 1.0 percent of body weight per week; losing weight too fast can significantly increases your risk for muscle loss and binge-like behaviors.

- The optimal weigh-in frequency for most is 2 – 3 times per week. As little as one time per week may not provide enough accurate information to assess progress and may also lead to disordered eating behaviors. Weighing in too often may also lead to disordered eating behaviors and an overdependence on the scale as an indicator of progress.

CHAPTER 12: WIN THE WEEKEND

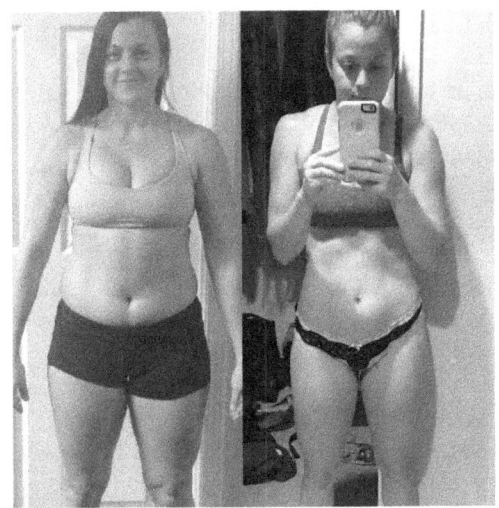

Anne Marie lost 18 pounds in 12 weeks!

Monday through Friday you crush it.

You're up at 6:00 a.m., hit the gym at 5:30 p.m., and in bed by 10:30 p.m. (let's exclude Friday from this latter part). You also eat five meals per day, many, if not all, of which, are prepped ahead of time. But as soon as the clock hits 5:00 p.m. on a Friday, all hell breaks loose.

It starts Friday night, when you stay up a few hours later than usual.

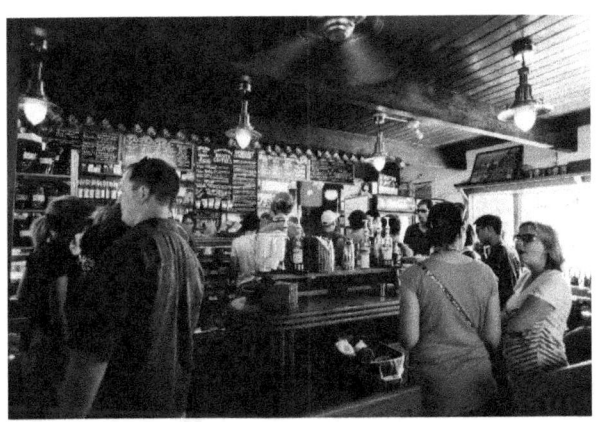

Does Friday night start your path to diet destruction?

Then, come Saturday morning, you have no reason to wake up at 6:00 a.m. Instead, you wake up when you wake up, which is often well past 9:00 a.m. And since there's no need to rush out the door, your usual five-minute shower becomes a 20-minute shower.

Furthermore, with no boss hovering over your shoulder, you're not confined to only five minutes on Facebook, and instead, can scroll leisurely, which typically lasts at least 20 minutes.

Finally, come 10:30 a.m. you decide you should get a move on making breakfast.

Instead of being locked into a routine for the next 12 hours, you have an open slate of possibilities. Sure, you'll get to the gym, at some point, but if you want to Netflix for a few hours, you can, and you will. And if you're like most people, you have zero meals prepped for the weekend, and probably little food in the fridge, too; thus, you plan to eat out for a meal—or three. And when you get home from dinner you stay up late again, well, just because you can. You don't have an alarm set and have no obligations early Sunday morning.

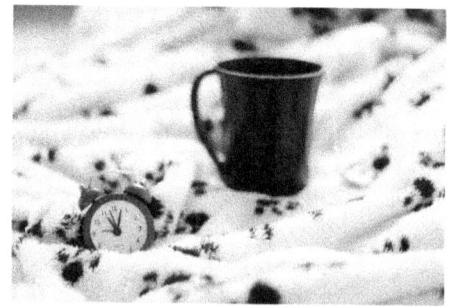

A warm blanket, warm beverage, and no obligations
makes it tough to stay in your routine on the weekends.

Do you see why many people take a step backwards during the weekend?

The result of a lack of structure leads to **taking two steps backwards**. This has a profound impact on progress.

Think about it: If you hit your goals 100 percent Monday – Friday, you take five steps in the right direction. If you're off track both Saturday and Sunday, however, it's as if you've taken two steps backwards, netting a total of three steps in the right direction. Had you been prepared to tackle the weekend you could have wound up with a **net of seven steps in the right direction**.

By taking the necessary steps to **win the weekend**, you can optimize your fat-loss progress!

Restructuring the Day

A change in your daily structure leads to missed meals and overcompensation later, eating out of boredom, or a combination of both. Either way, your nutrition is thrown out of whack. To overcome this change in structure, and avoid having it derail your dieting efforts, you need to prepare ahead of time.

For starters, **make** (notice I didn't say "take") time on either Thursday or Friday evening to prepare food for the weekend. Now, given that you may have a varying schedule, and may end up with last second plans, I encourage you to cook food in bulk, rather than to portion out individual meals.

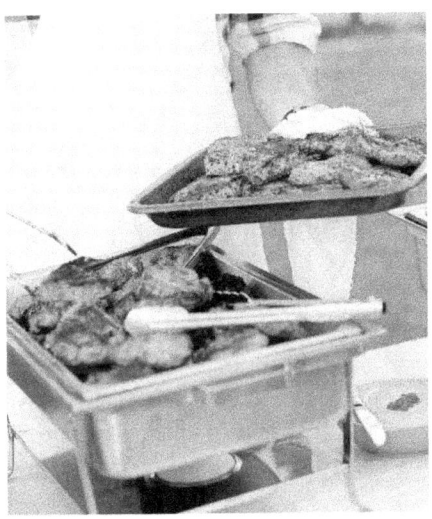

Cooking in bulk for the weekend is an excellent strategy to stay on track over the weekend.

By cooking lean protein and healthy carbohydrates in bulk, and of course, having ample vegetables on hand, you'll be able to quickly throw together a meal, while still being able to toggle with portions as needed.

Cooking in bulk rather than portioning out individual meals promotes flexibility for you to adapt to the day and adjust portions as necessary.

Furthermore, have plenty of high-protein, healthy snacks on hand that you can throw in a bag, purse, or your car and take with you to tackle a fun-filled day. Convenient, travel-friendly snacks include: whey/casein protein, Quest protein bars, Quest protein chips, beef jerky, lean deli meat, low-fat Greek yogurt, oats, fruit, nuts, seeds, nut butters. This can be a difference maker because if your afternoon activity runs long, you'll be able to still get some form of food into your body, which will lessen the likelihood of bingeing at a nearby restaurant later.

To make both above strategies possible for you to implement, you need to have a successful grocery trip. Whether that means making your weekly grocery trip on Thursday or Friday, replenishing staple snack items often, and stocking your freezer with protein every chance you get, you need to make it happen.

Navigating Social Occasions

Aside from a change in structure, the next biggest deterrent from your dieting efforts is having a social life. Whether you're attending a sporting event, concert, night out with friends, or hosting a family game night, I can guarantee that food will be the focus at some point. This makes many uneasy, and makes meeting calorie goals quite challenging.

Fortunately, by implementing some of the strategies you've learned in this book, you can be well on your way to a successful night of balancing food and fun. To further combat these special circumstances, implement one, or all, of the strategies below:

- **Exercise Before**- This will lessen the chance of straying significantly from your total planned calorie deficit for the day. Eating in excess and not exercising is far from ideal to continue making progress. If you think you may be a bit over on calories for the day, at least put those calories to good use (in support of muscle growth and recovery) by exercising prior.

- **Eat Before**- Have a protein-rich snack an hour before to help curb your appetite. This will help you save on calories and dollars.

- **Preload the Event with Water**- You should be drinking water frequently throughout the day anyway, but it's a great idea to drink even more before and during the event to keep hunger and temptation in check.

The best piece of advice I have for you: Treat the occasion like any other meal. What I mean by this is employ all the strategies you've learned so far at this one specific event. Prioritize protein, healthy carbohydrates, and vegetables; shift calories in favor of having more later in the day; eat every few hours; avoid alcohol. These strategies work in and out of a vacuum and are effective in multiple realms!

Dieting While Dining Out: Restaurant-Specific Strategies

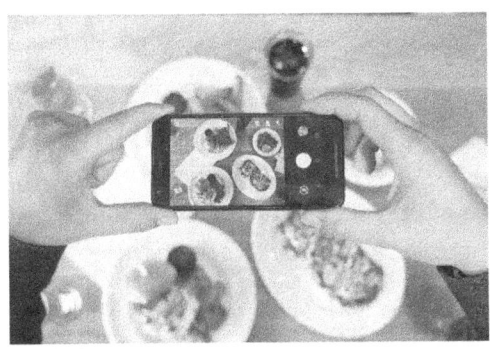

It's the chef's job to add anything and everything to make the food taste so delicious that you continue coming back again and again.

You can dine out and still lose weight. Although I don't encourage you to do it too often while dieting, it will inevitably happen, and can be a great break from meal prep, and even greater escape to spend time with loved ones.

It's important to remember that the goal of every restaurant chef is to make the food they serve taste as good as possible. If you love the meal, you'll come back for more, and ultimately, they'll make more money. Everyone wins.

What's the best way to enhance the flavor of a dish? Using copious amounts of butter, oil, and sugar, of course!

Unfortunately, this leads to many restaurant dishes being loaded in calories. Even smaller portions and certain salads can close in on one-thousand calories. This can make dieting while dining out tough. But if you follow the strategies below, you'll be able to stay well within limits of your goals for the day.

.
1. **Check the Menu Ahead of Time**- Most restaurants have their menus online. By reviewing it ahead of time, and seeking out the best option for you and your goals, you leave less chance of being swayed into choosing a less-than-optimal option for your goals when you've succumbed to the aromas and pretty plates of food once inside the restaurant.

2. **Bypass the Bread (or Chips)**- Remember, restaurants want to keep you coming back again and again. One strategy they use to do this is to make sure you enjoy every part of the experience. What's more enjoyable: waiting for your food and being forced to talk to your company, or, waiting for your food, being forced to talk to your company, AND having the option to snack in the meantime?

   Hopefully, you enjoy both, but having some warm bread, or crunchy chips, can make any experience better. Unfortunately, this situation usually entails mindless eating of calorie-dense foods, which can add up quickly and negate your hard work for the day...or days past. Kindly ask your server not to bring any out if your company is fine with it. Or, don't put a plate in front of you and keep the basket out of arm's reach.

3. **Drink Water**- It's calorie free and doesn't cost a dime. It also keeps appetite in check. Need any other reasons to stick to water? Diet beverages are A-Okay, too.

4. **Start with a Salad**- Start your meal with a salad to get a jump-start on sending satiety signals to your brain. An array of vegetables will help to fill your stomach, and make sure that by the time you finish your smaller portion dinner you are indeed mentally and physically full.

   Be sure that your salad is comprised of a variety of different colored vegetables, and not loaded with cheese, croutons, bacon, eggs, etc. A little bit is fine, but the point of this salad is to have low-calorie vegetables to occupy space in your stomach. The additional toppings can send calories skyrocketing in a heartbeat. Ask for the dressing to be served on the side and use in moderation only as needed.

5. **Order a Lean Protein and Vegetable**- Both items work to slow digestion and promote fullness. Make them the focal point of your meal. If you do plan to order a carbohydrate-containing entrée, I encourage you to focus on eating your protein and vegetable first, so that you're fairly full by the time you do get to your carbohydrate. This will lessen the chance of you mentally wanting more food, and picking at your dinner partner's portions!

6. **Ditch Dessert**- This should go without saying, but save the money and calories and ask for the check as you finish up your entrée.

Bonus Strategy: Eat Fewer Meals

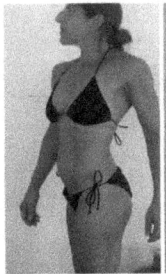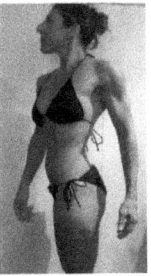

To help navigate a busy schedule, change in daily structure, and increase in temptations, consider eating fewer meals. By choosing to eat less frequently, you allot for larger portions at each feeding period. This will ensure you're mentally and physically full each time you eat, which will reduce cravings, as well.

Furthermore, it will alleviate then mental burden of striving to eat every three hours when you have commitments throughout the day. By doing so, you can relax and know that you can eat within three to five hours as your schedule permits.

If you typically eat five to six meals per day, consider reducing to four meals per day. Once you make this change, increase protein per meal by one to two ounces, and spread your carbohydrates and fats evenly throughout the day, making sure you have ample carbohydrates at your pre- and post-workout meals. And don't forget to have veggies at each meal!

Sample: 6 meals per day

Meal #	Protein (g)	Carbohydrates (g)	Fat (g)	Veggies (one handful)
Meal 1	24	15	15	1
Meal 2	24	25	10	1
Meal 3	24	40	5	1
Meal 4	24	60	5	1
Meal 5	24	30	10	1
Meal 6	24	10	15	1
Total	144	200	60	6

Sample: 4 meals per day

Meal #	Protein (oz.)	Carbohydrates (g)	Fat (g)	Veggies (one handful)
Meal 1	36	40	15	1
Meal 2	36	50	15	2
Meal 3	36	60	15	2
Meal 4	36	50	15	1
Total	144	200	60	6

Chapter 12 Recap:

- The weekend represents a major change in structure and routine. Failure to go in with a plan can lead to taking two steps in your diet, netting you a total of three positive steps for the week, rather than seven.

- Prepare food in bulk and advance to give yourself the opportunity to eat conveniently on the fly to adapt to an ever-changing weekend schedule.

- Consider reducing the number of meals you eat per day on the weekends to account for a change in schedule, more food availability, e.g., social gatherings revolving around food, and less time spent awake (related to sleeping in).

- Make exercise a priority on the weekend to help keep your total calorie balance in line with your goal of achieving a calorie deficit.

CLOSING THOUGHTS

Over the last 12 chapters, I've discussed what I've found to be the most impactful tips to apply to a dieting phase to create the best outcome. It's important to note, however, that dieting will still leave you hungry and feeling fatigued even if you implement the 12 tips discussed. This is because dieting is a major stress to your body. And quite frankly, if losing weight and keeping it off was easy, America wouldn't have a obesity epidemic on its hands.

My hope is that after reading this book, you find a few tips that you've yet to implement to past diets, and by implementing said tips to your next diet, hunger and fatigue are a little less noticeable, and that you're able to push through until the end. The results will not only be physically rewarding, but mentally, too, as you learn just how capable you really are.

As I blatantly stated in chapter 10, this book contains an underlying message of "be optimal." If you're sick of having little to no success losing weight and keeping it off, it's time to dig deep and ask yourself whether you've given your best effort in the past. Implementing these 12 tips can put you in a position to lose the weight you desire, and regain your health, confidence, and body back that being overweight has robbed you of.

Thank you for having enough belief in me to spend your hard-earned money on this book. It means a lot to me. My goal has always been to provide people with the information, tools, and confidence they need to eat healthily and confidently for life. I'm hopeful you'll find this book a staple source of all three.

Yours in health,

Paul J. Salter

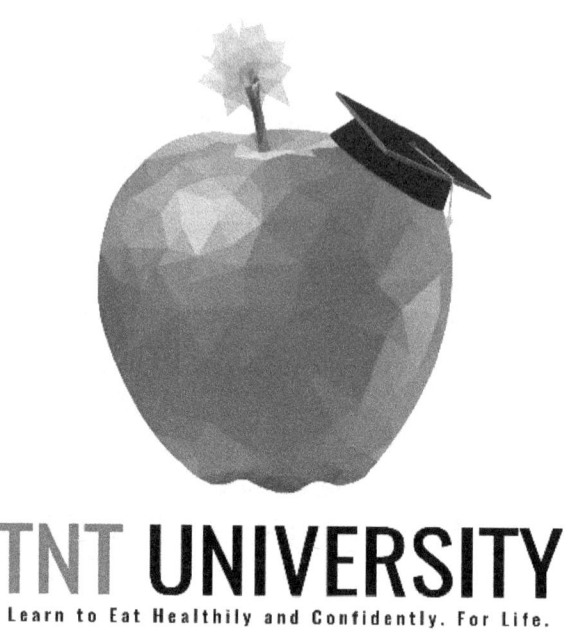

TNT UNIVERSITY
Learn to Eat Healthily and Confidently. For Life.

TNT University is your home for premiere online nutrition video courses. Each course details the need to know information on a variety of major nutrition topics. And even better, each video only lasts 2 – 5 minutes, making it easy for you to pay attention, learn, and get on with your day. By becoming a member of the TNT University Tribe, you also gain exclusive access to the TNT University private Facebook Group, which offers not only further learning, laughing, and support, but also access to private video Q&A and early product releases by me.

Visit:

https://courses.nutritiontactician.com/plans-and-pricing/

Here's what some of the Tribe members are saying about TNT University:

"Working with Paul was amazing — he was integral to the success I had. He's so great at educating...he helped me understand the 'why' of nutrition changes we made. I'm so grateful for working with Paul — he completely changed my life."

- **Kaitlin M.**

"I do love how each video in the carb course is short. It keeps me attentive and wanting to keep clicking to the next video, but is also a good way to not lose track of your progress when you don't have much time to finish everything. Thanks again!"

- **Jayne J.**

"I wanted to say thank you for your Carbs course. I'm a Personal Trainer and Nutrition Consultant. I have been in business 7 years now and following RP & JTS for about 3-4 years now. I decided to refresh my knowledge on the topic with TNT University. I was happily surprised to see the format of your educational content. It's brilliant, simple and straight to the point. Bravo. Merci beaucoup!!! I look forward to (re)learning more soon."

- **Sebastien L.**

REFERENCES

Chapter 1: Prioritize Protein

1. Belza, A., Ritz, C., Sørensen, M. Q., Holst, J. J., Rehfeld, J. F., & Astrup, A. (2013). Contribution of gastroenteropancreatic appetite hormones to protein-induced satiety. The American Journal of Clinical Nutrition, 97(5), 980-989.

2. Halton, T.L. & Hu, F.M. (2004). The Effects of High Protein Diets on Thermogenesis, Satiety and Weight Loss: A Critical Review. Journal of the American College of Nutrition, 23(5), 373-385.

Chapter 2: Choose High-Fiber Carbs

1. Phillips, R. J., & Powley, T. L. (1996). Gastric volume rather than nutrient content inhibits food intake.American Journal of Physiology-Regulatory, Integrative and Comparative Physiology, 271(3), R766-R769.

2. Wanders, A. J., van den Borne, J. J., de Graaf, C., Hulshof, T., Jonathan, M. C., Kristensen, M., ... & Feskens, E. J. (2011). Effects of dietary fibre on subjective appetite, energy intake and body weight: a systematic review of randomized controlled trials. Obesity Reviews, 12(9), 724-739.

Chapter 4: Hydrate, Hydrate, Hydrate

1. Kraft, J. A., Green, J. M., Bishop, P. A., Richardson, M. T., Neggers, Y. H., & Leeper, J. D. (2010). Impact of dehydration on a full body resistance exercise protocol. European Journal of Applied Physiology, 109(2), 259-267.

2. Judelson, D. A., Maresh, C. M., Farrell, M. J., Yamamoto, L. M., Armstrong, L. E., Kraemer, W. J., ... & Anderson, J. M. (2007). Effect of hydration state on strength, power, and resistance exercise performance. Medicine and Science in Sports and Exercise, 39(10), 1817.

Chapter 5: Eat Bland Food

1. Cabanac, M., & Johnson, K. G. (1983). Analysis of a conflict between palatability and cold exposure in rats. *Physiology & behavior, 31*(2), 249-253.

2. Oswald, K. D., Murdaugh, D. L., King, V. L., & Boggiano, M. M. (2011). Motivation for palatable food despite consequences in an animal model of binge eating. *International journal of eating disorders, 44*(3), 203-211.

3. Wise, R. A. (2006). Role of brain dopamine in food reward and reinforcement.*Philosophical Transactions of the Royal Society of London B: Biological Sciences, 361*(1471), 1149-1158.

4. Wise, R. A. (2004). Dopamine and food reward: back to the elements.*American Journal of Physiology-Regulatory, Integrative and Comparative Physiology, 286*(1), R13-R13.

5. Rolls, B. J., Rowe, E. A., Rolls, E. T., Kingston, B., Megson, A., & Gunary, R. (1981). Variety in a meal enhances food intake in man. Physiology & Behavior, 26(2), 215-221.

6. Rolls, B. J., Rowe, E. A., & Rolls, E. T. (1982). How sensory properties of foods affect human feeding behavior. Physiology & Behavior, 29(3), 409-417.

7. Pliner, P., Polivy, J., Herman, C. P., & Zakalusny, I. (1980). Short-term intake of overweight individuals and normal weight dieters and non-dieters with and without choice among a variety of foods. Appetite, 1(3), 203-213.

Chapter 7: Eat Every 3 – 5 Hours

1. Norton, L. (2008). Optimal protein intake and meal frequency to support maximal protein synthesis and muscle mass. JISSN, 3(5), S4.

2. Rennie, M. J., Bohé, J., & Wolfe, R. R. (2002). Latency, duration and dose response relationships of amino acid effects on human muscle protein synthesis. The Journal of Nutrition, 132(10), 3225S-3227S.

3. Diabetes Management: From Today´s Standards to Tomorrow´s. On the occasion of the Annual Meeting of the EASD, Copenhagen, Denmark (2006). Accessed September 14, 2016. Retrieved from: http://www.diabetes-symposium.org/index.php?menu=view&chart=4&id=322.

4. Juvenile Diabetes Research Foundation Continuous Glucose Monitoring Study Group. (2010). Variation of interstitial glucose measurements assessed by continuous glucose monitors in healthy, nondiabetic individuals. *Diabetes Care*, *33*(6), 1297-1299.

Chapter 10: Avoid Alcohol

1. Bullock, C. (2010). The Biochemistry of Alcohol Metabolism—A Brief Review. Biochemical Education, 18(2), 62-66.

Chapter 11: Don't Relay On The Scale

1. Heckerman, C.L., Brownell, K.D. & Westlake, R.J. (1978). Self and external monitoring of weight.*Psychological Reports*, *43*(2), 375-378.

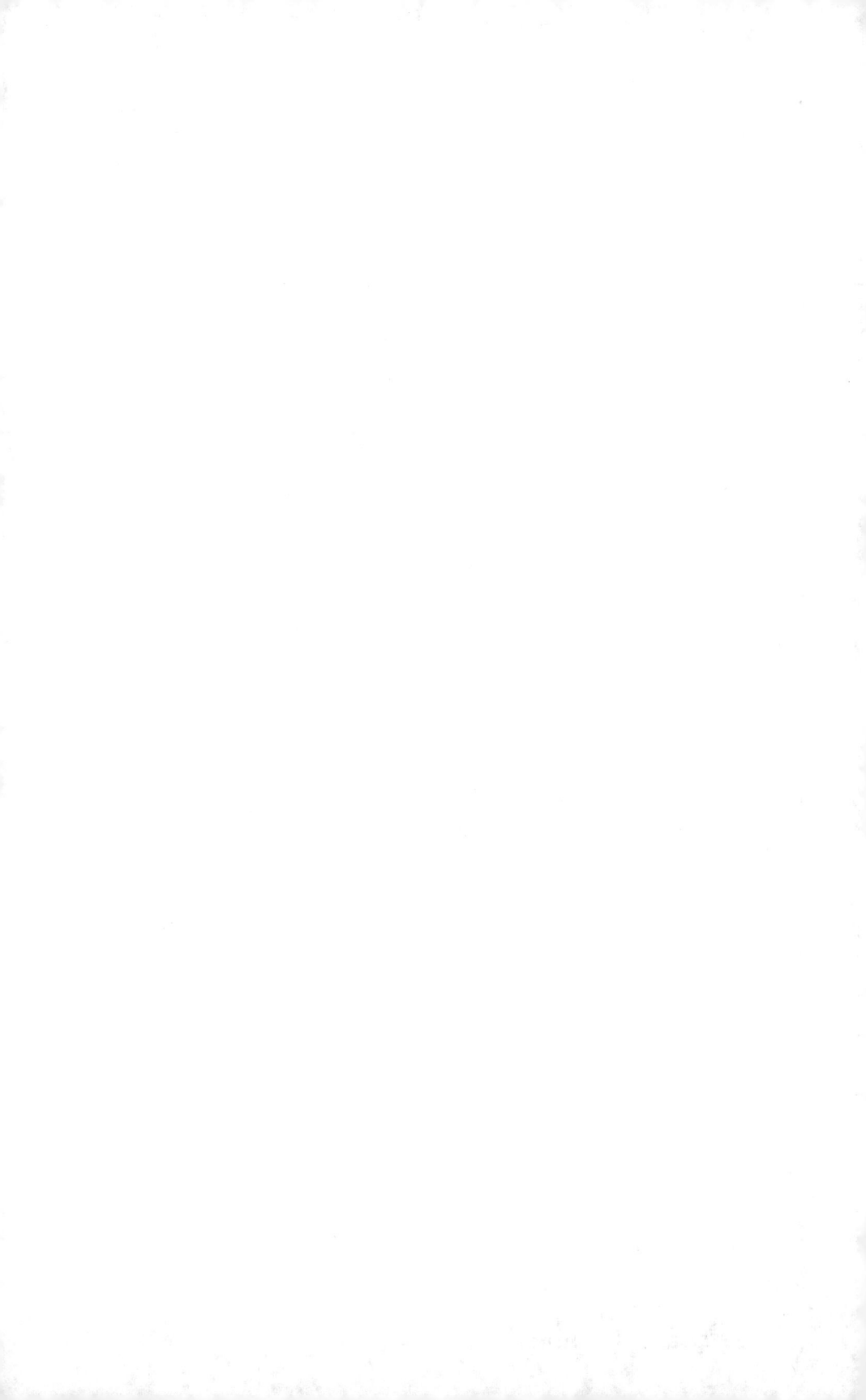

www.ingramcontent.com/pod-product-compliance
Lightning Source LLC
Chambersburg PA
CBHW072101280526
45788CB00006B/2354

* 9 7 8 1 5 4 2 6 4 0 9 6 1 *